SARS, Governance and the Globalization of Disease

Also by David P. Fidler

ROUSSEAU ON INTERNATIONAL RELATIONS (*Stanley Hoffmann and David P. Fidler, eds*)

EMPIRE AND COMMUNITY: EDMUND BURKE'S WRITING AND SPEECHES ON INTERNATIONAL RELATIONS (*David P. Fidler and Jennifer M. Welsh, eds*)

INTERNATIONAL LAW AND INFECTIOUS DISEASES

INTERNATIONAL LAW AND PUBLIC HEALTH: MATERIALS ON AND ANALYSIS OF GLOBAL HEALTH JURISPRUDENCE

STEALING LIVES: THE GLOBALIZATION OF BASEBALL AND THE TRAGIC STORY OF ALEXIS QUIROZ (*Arturo J. Marcano Guevara and David P. Fidler*)

SARS, Governance and the Globalization of Disease

David P. Fidler

Professor of Law and Ira C. Batman Faculty Fellow, Indiana University, USA

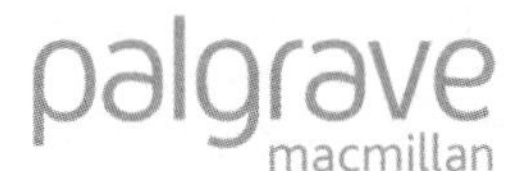

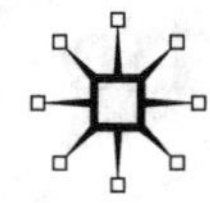

First published 2004 by
PALGRAVE MACMILLAN
Houndmills, Basingstoke, Hampshire RG21 6XS and
175 Fifth Avenue, New York, N.Y. 10010
Companies and representatives throughout the world

PALGRAVE MACMILLAN is the global academic imprint of the Palgrave Macmillan division of St. Martin's Press, LLC and of Palgrave Macmillan Ltd. Macmillan® is a registered trademark in the United States, United Kingdom and other countries. Palgrave is a registered trademark in the European Union and other countries.

ISBN 1–4039–3326–X

This book is printed on paper suitable for recycling and made from fully managed and sustained forest sources.

A catalogue record for this book is available from the British Library.

Library of Congress Cataloging-in-Publication Data
Fidler, David P.
SARS : governance and the globalization of disease / David P. Fidler.
p. cm.
Includes bibliographical references and index.
ISBN 1–4039–3326–X (cloth)
1. SARS (Disease)—Government policy.
2. SARS (Disease)—Epidemiology. I. Title.

RA644.S17F53 2004
614.5'92—dc22

2003070257

10 9 8 7 6 5 4 3 2 1
13 12 11 10 09 08 07 06 05 04

Printed and bound in Great Britain by
Antony Rowe Ltd, Chippenham and Eastbourne

To the members of the Department of Communicable Disease Surveillance and Response, World Health Organization, who led the successful global campaign against SARS

Contents

Tables and Figures

Tables

Figures

Foreword

The outbreak of Severe Acute Respiratory Syndrome (SARS) in 2003 and its successful global containment are testimony to a new way of working internationally for the public good. During the outbreak of SARS in 2003, I was the Executive Director of Communicable Diseases at the World Health Organization (WHO) and witnessed first-hand the events as they unfolded. David P. Fidler's book, *SARS, Governance and the Globalization of Disease*, wonderfully captures the historic nature of the SARS outbreak and the complexity and innovation of how this threat to global health security was detected and contained.

My career as an epidemiologist has permitted me to work on the control of infectious diseases that range from smallpox, Ebola and polio to AIDS, tuberculosis and malaria, since 1976. During these years, we have seen infectious diseases emerge and re-emerge, and threaten public health in all corners of the globe. The emergence of previously unknown infectious diseases, such as AIDS and Ebola, and the sudden appearance of diseases, such as West Nile virus infection, on new continents, combined with the increased speed and volume of international trade and travel, have made countries conscious of their vulnerability to new and emerging infectious disease threats that easily cross borders. In a globalized world, microbes travel freely from continent to continent in humans, often without any symptoms during the incubation period. They also travel in insects, livestock, and food and are able to infect humans in transit or at their final destination. As Professor Fidler explains, SARS emerged into this threatening context and reinforced the mutual vulnerability of societies to microbial threats.

A high proportion of new and emerging infectious diseases come from developing countries, often those least equipped to detect and respond to them early, and to contain them before they spread internationally. But all countries are vulnerable to outbreaks either because they emerge within national borders or present external threats through international spread. Decreased investment in public health – a problem that had reached crisis proportions by the 1960s and 1970s – has increased such vulnerability. For decades, both national budgets and international development agencies shifted resources to priorities other than public health, partially because of a growing and misplaced optimism that new antibiotics and vaccines would keep infectious diseases under control.

The rapid international spread of AIDS in the 1980s tempered this optimism and called attention to the need for increasing resources for public health, and for a global alert mechanism that could identify and effectively respond to infectious disease outbreaks that threatened to spread internationally. With the intentional release of anthrax to cause harm and incite terror in the United States, and the concerns this incident raised internationally, microbial agents are now more than ever perceived as a clear and present danger to public health security nationally and globally. At the same time, greater investment in public health defences against naturally occurring emerging infections, including strong global alert and response mechanisms, contributes powerfully to the detection of, and public health response to, outbreaks that might be deliberately caused. As Professor Fidler analyses, questions concerning the framework for detection of infectious disease outbreaks and the coordination of the international response – what he rightly calls the governance of infectious disease outbreaks – became a central question both within and among states during the 1990s.

When SARS began to spread internationally in February 2003, detection and a coordinated international response were possible because one such governance investment in global surveillance had already been initiated. The WHO-coordinated Global Outbreak Alert and Response Network (GOARN), which first detected SARS and facilitated the global response, was set up in 1997 and formalized in 2000 to improve global health security in a time of increasing microbial threats. GOARN is a network of over 120 partner networks for surveillance, disease detection, and public health response that covers the world. Each year, GOARN detects and mounts a coordinated international response to over 50 outbreaks, mainly in developing countries, that range from cholera and meningitis to yellow fever, plague, and Ebola. GOARN serves as a global safety net by reinforcing national surveillance and response to infectious disease outbreaks, particularly in developing countries, and by protecting the world against the international spread of microbial dangers.

As Professor Fidler's book meticulously explains, GOARN was a catalyst for the successful containment of SARS. In February 2003, two months after having detected what was a confirmed influenza outbreak in the Guangdong Province of China in late 2002, GOARN partners detected and responded to an outbreak of highly fatal atypical pneumonia in Viet Nam; but experts soon ruled out influenza. The infection rapidly spread to health workers and their immediate contacts. By 12 March, GOARN had obtained enough information about the outbreak to prompt WHO to issue its first global alert about the new infectious disease spreading in Asia. By 15 March, further information from GOARN partners made it clear that the disease was spreading beyond Asia; and WHO issued a second global alert that named the disease, provided a case definition for public health authorities and clinicians, and alerted international travellers about the spread of the new disease. Thus began an unprecedented effort to coordinate a global response to the emergence and international spread of a new infectious disease, putting these new global health governance mechanisms to the test for the first time in an outbreak of intercontinental proportions.

Professor Fidler's book also concisely analyses other aspects that made the global containment of SARS possible. During the response to SARS, GOARN electronically linked some of the world's best laboratory scientists, clinicians, and epidemiologists in virtual networks that rapidly created and disseminated knowledge about the causative agent, mode of transmission, and other epidemiological features of SARS. By the time the outbreak had been fully contained, 152 experts from institutions in 17 different countries had responded at sites where the outbreak was under way and had provided real-time information that made it possible for WHO to provide specific guidance to health workers about clinical management and to public health authorities concerning interventions to prevent further spread.

As Professor Fidler properly highlights, these globally coordinated activities also made possible WHO's evidence-based recommendations to international travellers as part of the global effort to curtail the international spread of SARS. Recommendations were at first non-specific, urging international travellers to have a high level of suspicion if they had travelled to or from areas where the outbreak was occurring. As more information became available, airports were asked to screen passengers for possible contacts with SARS and for persons with current illness that fit SARS case definition. Finally, when these recommendations did not completely stop international spread, WHO asked passengers themselves to avoid travel to areas where contact tracing was unable to link all cases to known chains of transmission.

Partially because of the profound economic impact of SARS, partially because of the fear it had created among their citizens, heads of state, diplomats and politicians became involved early and visibly, fully participating in outbreak control through frequent press briefings, declarations, and provision of political and economic support to the global containment effort. Special meetings were held among ministers of health and heads of state of the APEC and ASEAN countries in order to enhance collaboration in control, and regional surveillance and response systems were designed and established as safeguards for future infectious disease outbreaks. And in some countries where the outbreak occurred, political leaders who did not contribute satisfactorily were replaced by others. Professor Fidler's book places great emphasis on the political context and dynamics of addressing not only SARS but also infectious diseases more generally.

Within four months of the recognition of the SARS outbreak, transmission of SARS had been interrupted in all affected countries. On 5 July 2003, WHO declared that the outbreak had been successfully contained. This accomplishment for global public health also established a foundation for future detection and response activities. By the time SARS was contained, the global effort had developed and placed in the public domain a comprehensive knowledge base about this newly identified human disease, which is available to the world's public health experts and scientists as they continue their surveillance, research activities, and preparations for additional outbreaks should they occur.

The management of the SARS outbreak is critical for the future of global infectious disease control in terms of global governance. The coordinated international response to SARS under GOARN followed a proposed new way of working under the International Health Regulations (IHR), the set of international legal rules that provide WHO its mandate for global infectious disease surveillance and response. The IHR seek to ensure maximum public health security in the face of the international spread of infectious diseases, but the Regulations have not kept pace with the nature of the microbial menace. The WHO Member States last significantly revised the IHR in 1969. They currently require reporting of three infectious disease – cholera, plague, and yellow fever – and set out pre-determined appropriate ways of responding to these diseases. Infectious threats in the world today include more than the three IHR target diseases; and, with electronic communications as used by GOARN partners, epidemiological information can be obtained to make real-time, evidence-based strategies and recommendations for outbreak responses, tailored to the challenges of each event and updated as necessary. In 1996, WHO began a revision process to update the IHR based on these observations. As Professor Fidler examines in detail, the global response to SARS demonstrated the power of this new way of working.

Following the World Health Assembly's adoption of a resolution on the IHR in May 2003, the revised IHR will hopefully permit WHO to take on a more forceful role in leading the fight against any infectious disease that threatens global health security. In a second resolution specific to SARS, the World Health Assembly asked countries to strengthen their disease surveillance and response mechanisms, to report cases promptly and transparently, and to provide any information requested by WHO that could help prevent further international spread. Across-the-board strengthening of national mechanisms for outbreak alert and response is the only rational way to defend public health security not just against SARS, but against all future infectious disease threats.

In the mid-nineteenth century John Snow, sometimes called the father of modern epidemiology, successfully controlled an outbreak of cholera in London by mapping the location of households where persons who had died from severe debilitating diarrhoea lived. With this map, Snow linked the outbreak to a water source on Broad Street in central London; and he directed health workers to remove the handle from the Broad Street water pump, forcing the use of an alternate water supply. Snow's analysis and intervention stopped the outbreak.

Though the intercontinental spread of SARS began on the single floor of a hotel, SARS control efforts coordinated through GOARN never faced an option so simple as removing a handle from a single pump. But, as more and more evidence accumulated through the global, real-time collaboration of public health experts, control measures were introduced to meet specific needs. Just as John Snow had done in London, GOARN used the epidemiological evidence to formulate interventions that stopped the outbreak. The willingness of the international community to form a united front against a shared threat in response to the SARS outbreak in 2003 may well become a milestone that shows how, in a closely interconnected and interdependent world, a new and poorly understood disease, with no vaccine and no effective cure, can be rapidly and effectively controlled.

Professor Fidler has written an accurate, accessible, and thought-provoking analysis of the SARS outbreak. The conceptual, historical, and political perspectives he applies to the SARS outbreak illustrate why the global public health response to this disease threat deserves wide-ranging consideration as the struggle with infectious diseases continues.

DAVID L. HEYMANN, M.D.

Special Representative to the Director-General of the World Health Organization for Polio Eradication, and formerly the Executive Director of Communicable Diseases at the World Health Organization

Preface

This book began its life as an article, 'SARS: Political Pathology of the First Post-Westphalian Pathogen,' which was published in the *Journal of Law, Medicine & Ethics* in the winter of 2003. I thank Lawrence O. Gostin, Professor of Law at Georgetown University and Professor of Law at Johns Hopkins University, and Director of the Center for Law and the Public's Health at Georgetown and Johns Hopkins Universities, for inviting me to write the article on SARS for this journal and, thus, providing me with a platform to conceive of this book. The ideas I developed in this book were sharpened in seminars and colloquia at Southern Illinois University School of Law, McGeorge School of Law at the University of the Pacific, and Indiana University School of Law at Bloomington; and I thank all those who participated in these intellectual endeavors and helped me refine and advance my ideas and arguments. I would also like to thank Cindy Buys, Leslie Gielow Jacobs, Gene Matthews, Tony Moulton, Rick Goodman, Nick Drager, Mary Kay Kindhauser, and David Heymann for their encouragement of my pursuit of this topic. Funding for my research on and writing of this book was generously provided by the Indiana University School of Law at Bloomington.

The book attempts to cover events concerning the SARS outbreak through the end of August 2003, when the manuscript was completed and submitted for publication. Even if, by the time this book is published, SARS has re-emerged, my hope is that it will still provide worthwhile scholarship and commentary on the historic meaning of the SARS outbreak of 2002–03 on the governance of infectious diseases in a globalized world.

D.P.F.

Abbreviations

AIDS	Acquired immunodeficiency syndrome
CISET	US National Science and Technology Council Committee on International Science, Engineering, and Techology
CDC	US Centers for Disease Control and Prevention
EIDs	emerging and re-emerging infectious diseases
GPGH	global public goods for health
GPHIN	Global Public Health Intelligence Network
HIV	human immunodeficiency virus
ICESCR	International Covenant on Economic, Social, and Cultural Rights
IHR	International Health Regulations
ILO	International Labour Organization
MNCs	multinational corporations
NGOs	non-governmental organizations
PAHO	Pan American Health Organization
PCIJ	Permanent Court of International Justice
SARS	Severe Acute Respiratory Syndrome
SARS-CoV	SARS-associated coronavirus
TRIPS	WTO Agreement on Trade-Related Aspects of Intellectual Property Rights
UN	United Nations
UNAIDS	Joint United Nations Programme on HIV/AIDS
US	United States of America
WHO	World Health Organization
WTO	World Trade Organization

1
Introduction: The Importance of the SARS Outbreak

The coughs heard round the world

On 21 February 2003, Liu Jianlun, a 64-year-old physician and medical professor from Guangdong Province in the People's Republic of China, checked into the Metropole Hotel in Hong Kong, Special Administrative Region of China. Dr Liu had traveled to Hong Kong to attend a wedding. The hotel assigned him a room on the ninth floor, Room 911. Before his journey to Hong Kong for the wedding, Dr Liu had been treating patients in Guangdong Province who were suffering from a mysterious respiratory illness. By the time Dr Liu arrived in his room on the ninth floor of the Metropole Hotel, he had started to feel unwell. Dr Liu was feeling feverish and had begun to cough.

The rest, as the old saying goes, is history. In this case, global public health history. Dr Liu's stay at the Metropole Hotel in Hong Kong seeded a global epidemic of a disease entirely new to human populations. Dr Liu's coughs spread a new virus, never before experienced by humans, into one of the world's most cosmopolitan and globalized cities. From Hong Kong, the new disease traveled to new destinations within and beyond Asia in the respiratory tracts of a growing number of people, who themselves became vectors for the transmission of a new plague. Dr Liu's coughs at the Metropole Hotel introduced the world to what became known as Severe Acute Respiratory Syndrome (SARS) and triggered a global public health emergency the likes of which the world had not experienced in the modern age of public health.

Dr Liu's coughing in the Metropole Hotel also helped the world discover, again, that humanity's battle with infectious diseases continues. Just over three decades before Dr Liu's trip to Hong Kong, the US Surgeon General declared that modern public health and medicine had finally conquered infectious diseases, freeing the energies and technologies of epidemiology, medicine, and science to wage war on the rising scourge of non-communicable diseases (Emerging Infections Hearings, 1995, p. 1). These triumphalist claims appeared to be the fulfillment of the conquest of infectious diseases predicted and anticipated by many public health experts for decades. For example, Charles-Edward Winslow argued in 1943 that the application of modern principles of public health, combined with the development of antimicrobial drugs, had 'forever banished from the earth the major plagues and pestilences of the past' (Winslow, 1943, p. 380).

In the 30 years since the US Surgeon General proclaimed victory over pathogenic microbes, infectious diseases have made, and continue, a frightening resurgence. So-called naturally occurring infectious diseases emerged and re-emerged in the last three decades at such a pace and volume that the World Health Organization (WHO) declared in the mid-1990s that the world was facing a global crisis with respect to pathogenic microbes (WHO, 1996, p. 105). Infectious disease problems have become legion. New diseases have arisen, one of which – HIV/AIDS – proceeded to become one of the worst disease epidemics in human history (UNAIDS, 2002b, p. 44). Old microbial killers, such as tuberculosis, malaria, and cholera, were gaining strength in the face of deteriorating public health systems, declining effectiveness of antimicrobial drugs, and the new opportunities globalization created for microbial traffic (WHO, 1999; Institute of Medicine, 2003). Infectious diseases prevalent mainly in developing countries – so-called 'neglected' diseases – continued to cause death and disability on a significant scale (*Médecins Sans Frontières*, 2001; WHO, 2002a, pp. 104–53).

In parallel with growing concerns about the revenge of the pathogens, fears about the malevolent use of microbes by rogue states and terrorist groups increased dramatically. As the twentieth century came to a close, the United States and other nations began to address the rising threat of biological warfare and biological terrorism. Public health officials and experts, whose efforts had long been neglected and under-funded, missed no opportunity to harness the worries about biological weapons and bioterrorism to the larger challenges the microbial world was throwing at humanity.

Thus, the twenty-first century began with infectious diseases, especially HIV/AIDS, being discussed as threats to fundamental human rights (Hunt, 2003), sustainable economic development (Commission on Macroeconomics and Health, 2001), and national security (National Intelligence Council, 2000; Ban, 2001; Brower and Chalk, 2003). The perpetuation of bioterrorism in the United States in 2001 only heightened concerns about the threats pathogenic microbes posed. Infectious diseases also factored into the formulation of grand strategy for US foreign policy in the form of the Bush Doctrine, or the 'axis of evil' as it was originally known. The Bush administration declared that the most serious national security threat facing the United States came from oppressive regimes that were pursuing or possessed weapons of mass destruction and that were supporting international terrorism (Bush, 2002; *National Security Strategy of the United States*, 2002). Fears that Iraq would share weapons of mass destruction, including biological weapons, with Al Qaeda and other terrorist groups, formed part of the *casus belli* for the United States in its March 2003 invasion of Iraq. These fears also spurred the formulation and attempted implementation of an unprecedented smallpox vaccination program in the United States, in case the virus modern public health had eradicated in human populations in the late 1970s should return in the form of a weapon.

Attention in the early twenty-first century on naturally occurring infectious disease was also intense. Driven primarily by the horrifying expansion of the HIV/AIDS pandemic, analyses of global infectious disease problems reflected the urgency of the situation. The Institute of Medicine's Committee on Emerging Microbial Threats in the 21st Century argued immediately before the crisis of SARS broke upon the world that humanity confronted the prospect of recurrent microbial 'perfect storms' – repeated convergences of epidemiological, economic, political, and ecological factors that allow pathogens to emerge, spread, and root themselves in human societies with often devastating effects (Institute of Medicine, 2003, pp. 21–2). In all the ferment, epidemiologists worried about what was around the microbial corner. What would Mother Nature hurl next at a world still unprepared for more killer microbes? Pandemic influenza perhaps represented the worst nightmare scenario in the area of natural infectious disease concern.

Into this unprecedented, ominous, and *angst*-ridden environment on infectious diseases, Dr Liu coughed the coughs that would eventually be heard around the world.

An epidemic of 'firsts'

The SARS outbreak produced 8422 cumulative cases world-wide with 916 deaths between 1 November 2002 and 7 August 2003 (WHO, 2003a) (see Table 1.1). Statistically, these figures pale in comparison with the number of infections and deaths caused annually by other infectious

Table 1.1 SARS cases by country, 1 November 2002–7 August 2003

Country or area	*Total SARS cases*
Australia	6
Brazil	1
Canada	251
China	5327
China, Hong Kong Special Administrative Region	1755
China, Macao Special Administrative Region	1
China, Taiwan	665
Colombia	1
Finland	1
France	7
Germany	9
India	3
Indonesia	2
Italy	4
Kuwait	1
Malaysia	5
Mongolia	9
New Zealand	1
Philippines	14
Republic of Ireland	1
Republic of Korea	3
Romania	1
Russian Federation	1
Singapore	238
South Africa	1
Spain	1
Sweden	3
Switzerland	1
Thailand	9
United Kingdom	4
United States	33
Vietnam	63
Total	**8422**

Source: WHO 2003a

diseases. For example, HIV/AIDS, tuberculosis, and malaria account for over 500 million infections annually and approximately six million deaths (WHO, 2002b). More broadly, Table 1.2 lists the ten leading infectious diseases in terms of deaths for 2001 in order to provide an

Table 1.2 Leading causes of death by infectious diseases world-wide in 2001

Infectious disease	*Rank*	*Estimated number of deaths*
Respiratory infections	1	3 871 000
HIV/AIDS	2	2 866 000
Diarrheal diseases	3	2 001 000
Tuberculosis	4	1 644 000
Malaria	5	1 124 000
Measles	6	745 000
Pertussis	7	285 000
Tetanus	8	282 000
Meningitis	9	173 000
Syphilis	10	167 000

Source: WHO 2002c

indication of the magnitude of other infectious disease problems. Compared with the morbidity and mortality caused by other infectious diseases, the SARS outbreak's numbers make this epidemic seem minor and perhaps not worthy of all the attention it has garnered.

Statistics do not, however, reveal the historical importance of the SARS outbreak of 2002–03. SARS became an epidemic of 'firsts' for the global community, which helps explain why the outbreak is historic in many regards. Scientifically, the SARS epidemic constituted the first time the causative agent behind SARS – a novel kind of coronavirus – was identified in human populations (Ksiazek *et al.*, 2003; Drosten *et al.*, 2003). As such, this SARS-associated coronavirus (SARS-CoV) and the disease it caused created many questions scientists had never confronted before, such as exactly how this pathogen caused morbidity and mortality in humans.

The novelty of SARS-CoV generated new medical questions that the health care community struggled to understand during the outbreak. How does a clinician diagnose SARS? What was the incubation period of SARS? How should SARS patients be treated, and what were the best ways to protect medical personnel and other patients from contracting this new disease?

National and international public health officials and practitioners also felt the epidemic of 'firsts' related to SARS. The emergence of new viruses in human populations is not, of course, a new phenomenon for public health. SARS did, however, force public health authorities into a situation they had not confronted in the modern era of public health: How does public health contain the spread of a new virus spread efficiently by respiratory means from person-to-person without any effective diagnostic, therapeutic, or vaccine technologies? Compounding this public health challenge were the forces of globalization, especially the speed and volume of global air travel. As WHO articulated, SARS represented the first severe infectious disease to emerge into the highly globalized world society of the twenty-first century (World Health Assembly, 2003a) and demonstrated 'dramatically the global havoc that can be wreaked by a newly emerging infectious disease' (WHO, 2003b, p. 2). The number of infections and deaths caused by SARS has to be viewed in the context of the nature of the global threat SARS presented, the lack of medical technologies available to deal with the threat, the fear SARS provoked in individuals and societies around the world, and the serious economic damage the outbreak caused to countries and industries.

The successful containment of SARS on a global basis also constitutes part of the epidemic of 'firsts' triggered by the emergence of SARS. Infectious disease epidemics that have been contained in the past have involved diseases that effectively burned themselves out, remained limited to a specific geographical context, or were susceptible to the application of antimicrobial drugs and vaccines. SARS exhibited none of these characteristics. The respiratory means of SARS transmission meant that the syndrome did not burn itself out because of a lack of efficient human-to-human transmission. Global air travel spread the SARS virus around the world, ensuring that this would not be an infectious disease confined to a particular geographical location. The lack of any effective diagnostic, therapeutic, and vaccine technologies for addressing the SARS threat meant that public health authorities could not draw on the arsenal of science as they had done in containing past infectious diseases. Thus, SARS posed a public health governance challenge the likes of which modern public health had not previously confronted.

SARS and the governance of global infectious disease threats

The epidemic of scientific, medical, public health, and governance 'firsts' flows into the main argument of this book: SARS represents the first infectious disease to emerge into a radically new and different global political environment for public health. This book explores the emergence of SARS into a context for the governance of global infectious disease threats unlike the governance frameworks in place during previous outbreaks. I argue that the SARS outbreak confirms a transition from old to new forms of public health governance and teaches lessons about this transition that are both exciting and sobering.

As a concept, 'governance' refers to how societies structure responses to challenges they face. Governance clearly involves government as part of the structuring process, but governance and government are not synonymous. Making these two concepts synonymous would effectively mean that governance does not exist in international relations because no world government exists. Relations between independent, sovereign states in a condition of anarchy exhibit governance in the absence of a central, supreme government. Even those who adhere to the bleak pessimism of *realpolitik* acknowledge a governance structure in international politics – the strong do what they can, and the weak suffer what they must.

This book's foremost interest concerns describing and explaining why the SARS outbreak represents a historic moment in the governance of global infectious disease threats. Governance approaches to such threats have been present since at least the mid-nineteenth century, and the book explores the governance framework that dominated in this area since that time. But, as the above descriptions of ferment in national and international policy on infectious diseases suggest, challenges to the status quo were mounting and new thinking was developing prior to the emergence of SARS. For purposes of this book, the importance of the SARS outbreak arises from the convergence of the scientific, medical, and public health 'firsts' generated by SARS and the new governance framework emerging from struggles with the globalization of infectious disease threats.

SARS as the first post-Westphalian pathogen

The book asserts that SARS is the world's first 'post-Westphalian' pathogen in order to highlight the importance of what occurred in this outbreak for governance of infectious disease problems. As explained later in the book, I use the concept of the Westphalian international system developed by international relations scholars to demarcate public health governance before and after SARS. The term 'Westphalian' derives from the Peace of Westphalia of 1648, the historic settlement that ended the Thirty Years' War in Europe. International relations scholars identify the Peace of Westphalia as a landmark moment because it not only ended a bloody, continent-wide war but also established the basic principles for the political structure upon which governance of subsequent international relations was grounded. As Christopher Harding and C.L. Lim (1999, pp. 5–6) observed, '[a]s an event in the history of international relations the Treaty of Westphalia symbolically indicated a sea-change in international organisation – the transition to a system of sovereign states, as sovereigns subject to no higher or competing authority and conveniently determining the number and character of their legal relations with each other.'

As the first post-Westphalian pathogen, SARS provides an excellent case study of the transition of public health governance on infectious diseases from the traditional Westphalian framework to something new. The SARS case study not only illuminates governance shifts in public health but helps highlight changes that may be occurring to the general structure and dynamics of international relations in the era of globalization. Thus, the importance of the SARS outbreak goes well beyond the world of public health to encompass world politics generally.

A political pathology of SARS

The book constructs a political pathology of SARS and analyzes its implications for the future. 'Pathology' means the study of the causes, processes, and consequences of disease. I want to take the pathology of SARS – as pathology is traditionally understood – and analyze the scientific, medical, and public health challenges SARS creates through a political lens. The political pathology of SARS attempted in this book is a study of the causes, processes, and consequences of the governance of this disease.

I construct the political pathology of SARS in two parts. First, the book analyzes the governance transformation beginning to develop with respect to international infectious disease control prior to the SARS outbreak (Part I). This part begins with an exploration of the public health cliché that 'germs do not recognize borders' and stresses the importance of analyzing not only the germs but also the borders in connection with governance of infectious diseases (Chapter 2).

The next step in constructing the political pathology concentrates on distinguishing 'Westphalian public health' from 'post-Westphalian public health' (Chapters 3 and 4). I utilize a case study of the International Health Regulations – the most important set of international legal rules on infectious disease control – to elucidate the transition starting to take place from Westphalian to post-Westphalian public health in the 1990s and early 2000s.

The second part of the political pathology of SARS involves analyzing the SARS outbreak and post-Westphalian public health (Part II). After a brief history of the SARS outbreak of 2002–03 (Chapter 5), I examine China's confrontation with the governance framework of post-Westphalian public health (Chapter 6). China was the epicenter of the SARS outbreak, so focusing on China's response and behavior is appropriate and essential in exploring the political pathology of SARS. The book then looks beyond China's experience for more general lessons SARS teaches about post-Westphalian public health (Chapter 7).

The analysis of the political pathology of SARS includes examination of some of the vulnerabilities in post-Westphalian public health exposed by the SARS outbreak (Chapter 8). Although the governance response to SARS was exciting and successful, the outbreak highlighted significant problems, weaknesses, and on-going threats that post-Westphalian public health governance cannot ignore but may not be able to handle effectively. The final chapter offers concluding thoughts on the importance of understanding the political pathology of the SARS outbreak and the governance developments witnessed in the containment of this epidemic.

This book was written during the final stages and in the immediate aftermath of the SARS outbreak of 2002–03. I have been keenly aware in writing this book of the dangers of detailed analysis so close in time to such historic events. By the time this book is published, SARS may have re-emerged and produced more evidence and challenges for the political pathology constructed in this book. Despite the on-going, dynamic processes involved in governance of global infectious disease threats, I believe recording and analyzing at this time the governance events triggered by SARS contain value for thinking about infectious diseases in the globalized world of the early twenty-first century. Whatever transpires from this moment forward will find the SARS outbreak, governance, and the globalization of disease intertwined.

Part I

Westphalian and Post-Westphalian Public Health

2
Of Germs and Borders

Pathogens without passports

In some respects, the epidemic of 'firsts' discussed in Chapter 1 is misleading. What transpired in the SARS outbreak has frequently happened in the past – a new pathogenic microbe emerged in humans, spread to other countries through international trade and travel, caused economic, political, and social disruption, and revealed weaknesses in, or the non-existence of, public health capabilities. The great cliché of infectious disease control – germs do not recognize borders – applies to earlier outbreaks as equally as it applies to SARS. Public health experts could be forgiven for experiencing *déjà vu* as the SARS outbreak unfolded.

The 'germs do not recognize borders' mantra of public health is a mantra for good reasons. The mantra has a timeless quality because it applies to the spread of infectious diseases in every time period of human history. No matter what system of borders existed, germs did not recognize them. Germs did not recognize the borders of the ancient Greek city-states, as illustrated by Thucydides' grim telling of the plague of Athens during the Peloponnesian War. The borders of great empires posed no barriers to the spread of pathogenic microbes, as the Roman, Aztec, Inca, British, and American empires discovered in their respective historical periods. The Black Death ripped through fourteenth-century Europe untroubled by feudal borders. Germs of all sorts – bacteria, viruses, fungi, parasites, and prions – have bypassed the boundaries created by the modern inter-state system that has dominated world politics from the seventeenth to the early twenty-first centuries.

In the same way, the emphasis on the 'forces of globalization' in analyses of emerging and re-emerging infectious diseases in the 1990s and early 2000s sometimes neglected to recall that the globalization of public health was not a new phenomenon. Factors associated with infectious disease resurgence in the last decade of the twentieth century, especially the increased speed and volume of international trade and travel, were key factors in infectious diseases becoming more fearsome in the nineteenth century. This timeless quality of the 'germs do not recognize borders' mantra perhaps suggests that germ globalization is permanent while the borders are the transitory phenomena.

Although virtually all germs have potential to bypass borders, some germs are more dangerous than others when they do not recognize borders. In the pantheon of pathogens, these particularly dangerous microbes have a special place because their pathological profiles mesh seamlessly with the processes of globalization, especially the movement of people, goods, and animal and insect vectors through the channels of global commerce, travel, and migration. The great disease scourges of human history, such as smallpox, malaria, measles, tuberculosis, plague, cholera, and yellow fever, have each exploited global trade and travel to wreak great suffering on humankind.

Various developments in public health practices (e.g., surveillance and response) and technologies (e.g., modern water and sanitation systems, antimicrobial drugs, and vaccines) gradually loosened the deadly grip each of the great pestilences once possessed. The story of these achievements could be described as a case of public health globalization blunting the effects of germ globalization. The germs went global, followed by successful public health practices and technologies. Public health's counter-globalization did not necessarily benefit all segments of society equally because developing countries generally lagged behind the developed world in reducing infectious disease morbidity and mortality. As the Institute of Medicine's Committee on Emerging Microbial Threats in the 21st Century observed, '[m]ost developing nations have not shared fully in the public health and technological advances that have aided in the fight against infectious diseases in the United States.... In developing countries, clean water is scarce; sewage systems are overwhelmed or nonexistent; the urban metropolis is growing exponentially as the global market expands and rural agricultural workers migrate to cities; and economic need, political conflict, and wars are displacing millions of people and creating growing refugee populations' (Institute of Medicine, 2003, p. 27).

In addition to the higher burden of infectious diseases suffered by the developing world, the HIV/AIDS pandemic represents a great stain on twentieth-century public health progress on infectious diseases. From its origins in the early 1980s, this pandemic has joined the ranks of the most devastating plagues in the pantheon of pathogens. At the end of 2002, 42 million people were living with HIV/AIDS; and 27.9 million people had died from AIDS since the beginning of the pandemic in the early 1980s (UNAIDS, 2002a, p. 3). UNAIDS (2002b, p. 44) concluded at the end of 2002 that '[t]wenty years after the world first became aware of AIDS, it is clear that humanity is facing one of the most devasting epidemics in human history.' Most of the global burden of HIV/AIDS falls on developing countries, with nearly 70 per cent of all people with HIV/AIDS living in sub-Saharan Africa (UNAIDS, 2002a, p. 6). Ominously, leading HIV/AIDS expert Richard Feachem (2003) argued that '[h]orrifyingly, the worst is still yet to come' in connection with the HIV/AIDS pandemic.

Traditional globalizable public health practices, such as sanitation, were not helpful against the epidemiology of HIV/AIDS. Counter-globalization through drugs or vaccines has proved enormously difficult in the case of effective antiretrovirals. *Médecins Sans Frontières'* Campaign for Access to Essential Medicines argues, for example, that, as of December 2002, only 300 000 HIV-infected people living in the developing world were receiving antiretroviral treatment, with half of this number living in only one country, Brazil (*Médecins Sans Frontières*, 2003a). Efforts to develop a safe and effective vaccine for HIV have also, to date, not succeeded, leading to calls for an expanded global AIDS vaccine effort (Klausner *et al.*, 2003). In light of these public health handicaps, a seamless interface with global human mobility meant that HIV/AIDS did not recognize borders in a particularly devastating way.

As a germ that also does not recognize borders, SARS represents one of the most dangerous new pathogens to emerge in the last three decades (WHO, 2003b, p. 2). The SARS outbreak was the first infectious disease epidemic since HIV/AIDS to pose a truly global threat. Other microbes that have emerged in the last 30 years have had limited capacity to threaten global public health because of inefficient human-to-human transmission (e.g., avian influenza, Nipah, Hendra, and Hanta viruses), dependence in part on food or insects as vectors (e.g., *Escherichia coli* 0157:H7, variant Creutzfeldt–Jakob disease, West Nile and Rift Valley fevers) or on specific geographical locations (e.g., *Neisseria meningitides* W135, Ebola, Marburg, and Crimean–Congo haemorrhagic fevers) (WHO, 2003b, p. 3).

In SARS, the world confronted a virus never before found in humans that was transmitted from person to person, that had a high fatality rate (around 14–15 per cent but over 50 per cent in persons over age 65), and against which public health practitioners and clinical physicians had neither adequate diagnostic technologies nor effective treatments or vaccines (WHO, 2003b, pp. 2–3). The last time the world confronted a virus with this disturbing profile was when HIV emerged in the early 1980s, and HIV triggered one of the worst epidemics in history.

As bad as HIV/AIDS became, especially for developing countries and sub-Saharan Africa in particular, public health experts were thankful that HIV was not transmitted by respiratory means. SARS is, however, transmitted from person to person by such means, giving SARS an epidemiological profile well suited to take advantage of the opportunities globalization offers for microbial traffic. Although SARS is not 'airborne HIV' because the fatality rate of SARS is less than the 100 per cent death rate from untreated HIV, SARS' morbidity rate and respiratory route of transmission brought back bad memories of other global viral killers – the 1918–19 influenza and smallpox – that wrought havoc upon humankind. Even though the respiratory transmissibility of SARS was less robust than influenza or smallpox, this pathogen's non-recognition of borders constituted a world-wide public health threat.

The politics of passports

Public health experts often chant the 'germs do not recognize borders' mantra to make the epidemiological case that countries have to cooperate in addressing infectious disease threats. This appeal to countries immediately brings those epidemiologically irrelevant borders back into the picture. Germs have the luxury of existing in a borderless environment. Humans do not have this luxury. Borders are critical human institutions because they demarcate the political spaces in which human societies exist and through which they interact.

In my wallet, I carry an increasingly dog-eared passport filled with stamps from government agencies from countries around the world. The pages of my passport record that I do not live in a borderless world. Unlike microbes, border authorities regulate me when I cross international boundaries. The passport itself, and each stamp imprinted in it, is a statement about the existence and the importance of borders to human societies. The passport and the stamps it bears also connect to fundamental norms of world politics, such as sovereignty, territorial integrity, international order, and the self-determination of peoples. Historically, peoples living without borders have often suffered at the hands of those more powerful. Do not attempt to persuade a Palestinian living in the West Bank or the Gaza Strip that he or she should not desire an independent state because globalization makes borders meaningless.

Germs are epidemiological phemenona. Passports are political phenomena. The politics of passports drive how human societies respond to the threats germs pose. The politics of passports mean that human responses to pathogenic threats cannot entirely ignore borders and their consequences in the way microbes do. Understanding why the SARS outbreak is historic involves comprehending not only the germ but also the borders the germ did not recognize. The political pathology of SARS developed in this book is interested in the borders – the political and governance structures – that SARS did not recognize.

Like all endeavors undertaken by human societies, public health reflects larger political structures and forces that shape how and why societies pursue public health objectives. For example, in the United States, federalism structures public health governance in a particular way (Gostin, 2000, pp. 25–59). Federalism creates political borders between federal and state governments on public health and many other areas. The Constitution reserves the bulk of public health power to the individual states, while granting the federal government the ability to act on public health through its enumerated powers, such as the authority to regulate interstate and foreign commerce. Germs no more recognize these borders than they recognize international borders. Federalism does not, however, disappear as the primary structuring device for public health governance in the United States simply because germs do not recognize the boundaries it creates.

The Institute of Medicine (1988, p. 1) defined 'public health' as 'what we, as a society, do collectively to assure the conditions in which people can be healthy.' As with most traditional definitions of public health, the 'we' in the Institute of Medicine's definition – the collective society at the heart of activity – refers to a single sovereign state. The history of infectious diseases not recognizing borders demonstrates that the collective society encompassed by public health activities includes the community of states, or what international relations scholars call the 'international society.'

As defined by Hedley Bull (1977, p. 13), an international society 'exists when a group of states, conscious of certain common interests and common values, form a society in the sense that they conceive themselves to be bound by a common set of rules in their relations with one another, and share in the working of common institutions.' The start of international diplomacy on infectious disease control in the mid-nineteenth century and the subsequent development of international treaties on infectious disease control and international health organizations indicate that sovereign states formulated infectious disease control as a common interest and value and pursued this goal by creating and operating common rules and institutions. The existing political structure of international politics adjusted to the emergence of infectious diseases as a diplomatic problem, as opposed to the rise of the germs transforming the political structure of international relations.

As with federalism's impact on public health governance in the United States, the underlying political distribution of jurisdiction and competency among sovereign states creates another structural context for infectious disease governance dependent on the existence of borders, both territorial and political. Although germs do not recognize borders, boundaries between countries remain central to the process of structuring political responses to infectious disease threats. As explained in Chapter 3, principles derived from the general structure and dynamics of inter-state relations determined how and why countries engaged in governance activities on infectious diseases from the mid-nineteenth century.

Pathogens within politics

The effort in this book to analyze the political pathology of SARS contains the message that responses to pathogenic microbes are deeply political. In earlier work, I attempted to analyze the reality of pathogens within politics through the lens of what I called *microbialpolitik* – the international politics of infectious disease control (Fidler, 1998; Fidler, 1999; Fidler, 2001a). The political pathology of SARS explored in this book is a new and exciting chapter for *microbialpolitik* because of the way this outbreak reflected and accelerated changes in how pathogenic threats would be handled politically by states and other actors in international relations.

These changes are particularly important for *microbialpolitik* because, in many respects, the phenomenon of pathogens within politics has been fertile on the pathogens' side but static, or even stagnant, politically. When HIV/AIDS and other pathogens emerged and spread during the last 30 years of the twentieth century, the governance tools and approaches for responding to these challenges remained essentially the same as those first used in the mid-nineteenth and early twentieth centuries when infectious diseases first became a subject for diplomacy. Improvements in national public health capabilities and the development of antimicrobial drug and vaccine technologies fit into the traditional governance framework without causing structural stress. Progress against infectious diseases was recorded by many countries, particularly developed countries, during most of the twentieth century, suggesting that the traditional structure of *microbialpolitik* was not entirely dysfunctional. The global triumph of smallpox eradication in the late 1970s also indicated that public health could take significant strides without challenging the underlying structure of international politics.

These observations do not suggest that all was well with the traditional pursuit of 'international health cooperation' in the period before emerging and re-emerging infectious diseases took center stage in the 1990s. Some new political and governance notions appeared, such as the human right to health (WHO, 1948, Preamble; International Covenant on Economic, Social, and Cultural Rights, 1966, Article 12), which involved re-thinking infectious disease politics at the international level. The continuing and sometimes growing disparities between health in the developed and developing worlds created tension and dissatisfaction, as revealed by the World Health Organization's Health for All initiative at the end of the 1970s (Declaration of Alma Ata, 1978). More broadly, some experts, such as Charles Pannenborg (1979, pp. 342–91), called for a 'New International Health Order' in which developed countries would bear more political, economic, and legal responsibilities for raising health standards in the developing world.

Rhetoric on the human right to health, Health for All activism, and demands for a New International Health Order did not, however, effect any changes in the structure and dynamics of *microbialpolitik* by the beginning of the 1990s. But, in the last decade of the twentieth century, the traditional governance framework experienced enormous pressure and stress from the resurgence of infectious diseases and other global public health problems. The World Health Organization came under considerable criticism for presiding over global public health calamities, including HIV/AIDS (Fidler, 2000, pp. 109–10). Emerging and re-emerging infectious diseases destroyed systemic complacency on pathogenic microbes the existing governance structure of international health never overcame. The only international legal rules on infectious disease control binding on WHO member states – the International Health Regulations (IHR) – only addressed the same three diseases (cholera, plague, and yellow fever) (IHR, 1969, Article 1) discussed at the first international sanitary conference in 1851 (Goodman, 1971, p. 46). Experts identified intergovernmental actors, such as the World Bank and the World Trade Organization, and non-state actors (e.g., multinational corporations and non-governmental organizations) as growing influences on the substance of international public health policies (Fidler, 2000, pp. 72–83). The processes of globalization increasingly became the target of analyses of the growing threat posed by infectious diseases (Institute of Medicine, 1992; US CDC, 1994; CISET, 1995; Garrett, 1995; Fidler, 1996; WHO, 1996; Fidler, 1997a; Fidler, 1997b; Yach and Bettcher, 1998).

Rather than politics rendering pathogens less threatening to human societies, microbes were making the deeply grooved patterns of international governance on infectious diseases increasingly irrelevant to creating the conditions in which states and their peoples could be more secure against microbial threats. In the face of this crisis in *microbialpolitik*, the world needed a political and governance renaissance. The next two chapters examine the path public health began to travel in an effort to create a political response worthy of humanity's powerful pathogenic antagonists.

3
Public Health and the Westphalian System of International Politics

Introduction

The political pathology of SARS tells a tale of transition for governance on infectious disease threats. This chapter focuses on the beginning of this journey in order to explain the traditional governance structure and dynamics that determined how and why infectious disease threats were handled internationally. I do not provide a comprehensive and detailed history of international cooperation on infectious diseases; such histories have already been written (Howard-Jones, 1975; Goodman, 1971). Rather, this chapter has a conceptual orientation designed to provide a simple yet accurate picture of public health governance within the Westphalian system of international politics. The case study on the International Health Regulations (IHR) helps put the conceptual analysis into a more concrete form.

The world according to Westphalia

As Chapter 1 mentioned, international relations scholars often identify the Peace of Westphalia of 1648 as the birth of the modern international political system. Jan Aart Scholte (2001, p. 20) argues that the Peace of Westphalia 'contains an early official statement of the core principles that came to dominate world affairs during the subsequent three centuries.' Although what we recognize as territorial nation-states began to develop before the seventeenth century, this emerging political reality suffered for not having an overarching set of principles to give the nascent structure solid grounding. The Thirty Years' War in Europe at the beginning of the seventeenth century reflected the absence of an agreed political framework. This bloody conflict flowed from the explosive mixture of power politics and religious zealotry as Catholic and Protestant powers battled for temporal and spiritual supremacy in Europe.

The Peace of Westphalia is famous for not only ending the Thirty Years' War but also how this settlement established a political structure for international politics that has endured for over three centuries. I describe the basic structure, principles, and dynamics of the world Westphalia created. After laying out the main characteristics of the Westphalian system of international politics, I analyze how public health arose as an issue in this system.

The Westphalian system

A 'system' is a group of interacting elements that form a collective entity. The Westphalian system comprises independent, territorial states interacting in a condition of anarchy (Harding and Lim, 1999, pp. 5–6). International relations scholars often refer to the Westphalian configuration as an 'international system,' defined by Hedley Bull (1977, pp. 9–10) as forming 'when two or more states have sufficient contact between them, and have sufficient impact on one another's decisions, to cause them to behave – at least in some measure – as parts of a whole.' States dominate the Westphalian structure and determine the nature of anarchy in which they interact (Scholte, 2001, p. 20). The Westphalian system constructs anarchy as 'international anarchy' because of the central ordering role states play.

In the Westphalian system, 'anarchy' does not mean political confusion, disorder, or chaos. Anarchy means that the units of the system – the states – do not share or recognize a common, supreme authority (Dunne and Schmidt, 2001, p. 143). The Westphalian structure deliberately fragments political authority and power among the states, rendering any kind of world government impossible. The choice of a structure based on the anarchical interactions of independent states made at the Peace of Westphalia and sustained thereafter reflects not only political facts on the ground but also the determination that other ways of structuring international politics, such as some form of world government, were less palatable because of their potential to produce war and disorder, as the continent had experienced in the religiously motivated war among Catholic and Protestant powers. Philosophers as distinct as Jean-Jacques Rousseau and Immanuel Kant in the eighteenth century dismissed notions of a central, supreme government for European states as both illusory and dangerous to human well-being (Rousseau, 1756; Kant, 1795).

Westphalian governance principles

The fragmentation of political authority among a group of states interacting in a condition of anarchy created the need for principles to guide governance of such anarchical relations. The Westphalian system itself represents a rejection of government in the form of a common, supreme authority; but it is not a rejection of governance. In fact, the Peace of Westphalia established a system of governance for international anarchy. Westphalian governance is based on some fundamental principles.

The central governance principle of the Westphalian system is sovereignty – the states reign supreme over their territories and peoples (Brownlie, 1998, p. 289; Scholte, 2001, p. 20). Sovereignty provides the governance anchor for Westphalian politics because it demarcates the boundaries for the exercise of political authority. Sovereignty does not mean that a state's exercise of sovereignty is unaffected by the actions of other states. After all, Westphalian politics constitute a system based on the assumption that the units interact and that such interactions influence the behavior of the units.

The principle of sovereignty does, however, establish the preconditions for the legitimacy of the exercise of political authority in the Westphalian system. Flowing from the principle of sovereignty is the second fundamental tenet of Westphalian governance – the principle of non-intervention. Because sovereignty means supreme power over territory and people, Westphalian governance frowns upon one state intervening into the domestic affairs of other states (Brownlie, 1998, pp. 293–4; Jackson, 2001, p. 43).

The United Nations Charter (1945, Article 2.7) contains the principle of non-intervention when it declares that '[n]othing contained in the present Charter shall authorize the United Nations to intervene in matters which are essentially within the domestic jurisdiction of any State or shall require the Members to submit such matters to settlement under the present Charter'. Deriving much of its power from the sovereignty principle, the rule on non-intervention means that a state is free to determine its own political, economic, religious, and cultural systems. The Declaration on Principles of International Law Concerning Friendly Relations and Cooperation Among States (1970, p. 42) states, for example, that '[e]very state has an inalienable right to choose its political, economic, social, and cultural systems, without interference in any form by another State.' The principle of non-intervention excludes a great deal of sovereign behavior from being the subject matter of state interaction.

With governance within states rendered off limits by the sovereignty and non-intervention principles, Westphalian governance involved managing state interactions in anarchy. International law plays a central role in this task of anarchical management. Because no supreme, central government or law-making body exists in the Westphalian system, rules to govern the interaction of sovereign states arise from the states themselves. International law is a Westphalian governance process through which the states create, and consent to be bound by, certain rules of behavior in connection with their anarchical interactions.

The nature of the governance process means that a state is free to exercise its sovereignty as it sees fit unless that state had consented to be bound by a rule of international law that regulated its behavior in the relevant context (Brownlie, 1998, p. 289). The *SS Lotus* case decided by the Permanent Court of International Justice (PCIJ) in 1927 famously expressed this dynamic of Westphalian governance (*SS Lotus*, 1927). This case involved a dispute between France and Turkey over Turkey's exercise of criminal jurisdiction over a French national. The Frenchman was the captain of a French vessel that ran into a Turkish ship on the high seas. The collision sank the Turkish ship, killing eight Turkish nationals. When the French vessel docked at Constantinople, Turkey instituted criminal proceedings against the French captain for his actions on the high seas that led to the collision with the Turkish vessel.

France complained about the Turkish assertion of jurisdiction over the French national, arguing that Turkey could exercise its jurisdiction in this case only if a rule of international law expressly permitted such exercise. Turkey countered that it could exercise its jurisdiction in the case unless a rule of international law expressly prohibited Turkey from doing so. The PCIJ agreed with the Turkish position that no rule of international law prevented Turkey from exercising criminal jurisdiction over the captain of the French vessel. In explaining its reasoning in the case, the PCIJ stated:

> International law governs relations between independent States. The rules of law binding upon States therefore emanate from their own free will as expressed in conventions or by usages generally accepted as expressing principles of law and established in order to regulate the relations between co-existing independent communities or with a view to the achievement of common aims. Restrictions upon the independence of States cannot therefore be presumed. (*SS Lotus*, 1927, pp. 69–70).

Ever since, the *SS Lotus* case has served as a classical illustration of how international law functions in Westphalian governance. As the holding in the *SS Lotus* case demonstrates, sovereignty remains unfettered unless states themselves have created rules of international law to regulate the exercise of their sovereignty in their mutual relations.

The combination of the principles of sovereignty, non-intervention, and consent-based international law gives Westphalian governance a particular structure and subject matter. First, only states are involved in governance. This situation does not mean that non-state actors, such as companies and merchants, had no influence on the development of inter-state relations. After all, key modes of state interaction are trade and commerce, which have always involved private enterprises and entrepreneurs. How such trade and commerce is managed is, however, determined by states under the Westphalian template.

Second, Westphalian governance predominantly addressed the mechanics of state interactions, such as diplomacy, war, and trade. Even traditional rules that involved the treatment of individuals, such as international law on minimum standards of treatment of foreign nationals, connected to the interactions of states. The principles of sovereignty and non-intervention mean that Westphalian governance does not penetrate sovereignty to address how a government treats its people or rules over its territory. Governance in the Westphalian system is, thus, horizontal in nature because it occurs only between states and addresses issues raised by the interactions of states in the condition of anarchy (see Figure 3.1).

The politics of Westphalian governance

The structure and principles of Westphalian governance exhibit political characteristics that are important to describe. Under international law,

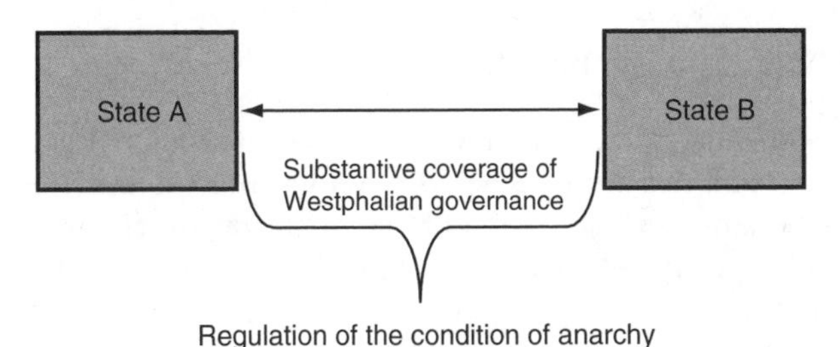

Figure 3.1 Horizontal governance

all sovereign states have equal standing in the formal functioning of the international legal system. As Brownlie (1998, p. 289) commented, '[t]he sovereignty and equality of states represent the basic constitutional doctrine of the law of nations, which governs a community consisting primarily of states having a uniform legal personality.' The United Nations Charter (1945, Article 2.1) reflects this doctrine in proclaiming that '[t]he Organization is based on the principle of the sovereign equality of all its Members.' The politics of Westphalian governance are not, however, egalitarian. The great powers have historically dominated and controlled the politics of the Westphalian system.

The leading role that great powers have played in the functioning of the international system has long been the subject of historical and theoretical analysis for international relations scholars. Histories of the development of international relations often focus on the machinations of the great powers because these states have initiated and shaped change in the system (e.g., Hinsley, 1963). The dominance of realism in international relations theory (Frankel, 1996, p. ix; Dunne and Schmidt, 2001, p. 145) also reflects the leading role of the great powers in Westphalian politics because realism focuses on the importance of possessing and exercising material power in the condition of anarchy that exists among states (Waltz, 1979, p. 131; Legro and Moravcsik, 1999, p. 18).

The old adage that power abhors a vacuum resonates in the Westphalian system. The anarchical environment in which sovereign states interact has historically placed a premium on having and using material capabilities, predominantly military and economic power, to ensure survival and the protection of national interests in the face of competition from other states. The states possessing the most power – the great powers – by and large have determined and controlled the substance and process of Westphalian governance, as illustrated by the dominant role the great powers had in the development of the modern system of international law (Nussbaum, 1954; Grewe, 2000).

Westphalian public health

The Westphalian structure and principles for international politics had been in place for two centuries before the cross-border spread of infectious diseases became a subject for international governance in the mid-nineteenth century. As Chapter 2 indicated, pathogens have been crossing borders since the beginning of human civilization; and they crossed borders established by the Westphalian system from the beginnings of this system in the mid-seventeenth century. The Westphalian system created, however, a particular governance structure and process through which states would address the international spread of infectious diseases.

Prior to the mid-nineteenth century, states in the international system handled infectious disease threats predominantly as a national issue and without systemic cooperation with other states. For example, European states adopted and implemented national quarantine measures in an effort to keep diseases from entering their territories from foreign lands. The practice of quarantines began in Italian city-states in the fifteenth century (Slack, 1992, p. 15); and, by the nineteenth century, 'nearly all civilized countries of the world adopted some form of quarantine control' (Goodman, 1971, p. 31).

Quarantine practices demonstrated that infectious diseases caused problems for the international system through state interactions fostered by trade and travel. In addition, the practice of requiring ships to acquire bills of health in order to avoid the application of quarantine measures illustrates the systemic impact of infectious diseases. A state would require that a ship, leaving a foreign port bound for one of its ports, obtain a bill of health stating that the ship's last port of call was free of epidemic diseases (e.g., plague, cholera, and yellow fever). The requiring state's diplomatic representative resident in the foreign country often had to certify bills of health to ensure their accuracy and legitimacy. Use of bills of health by states became widespread by the latter half of the seventeenth century (Goodman, 1971, p. 31).

Thus, diplomats were engaging in infectious disease control efforts long before the mid-nineteenth century. Yet, until the mid-nineteenth century, states attempted to handle the systemic effects of infectious disease transmission through the uncoordinated and unregulated exercise of national sovereignty. Quarantine measures and bills of health focused exclusively on preventing diseases from entering a state from foreign locations and relied exclusively on a nation's own governmental capabilities – diplomats abroad and quarantine officials at home. Westphalian governance on public health was, therefore, strictly a matter of sovereign discretion because of the absence of any international legal rules or diplomatic processes to manage the problem differently.

The growing threat of infectious diseases in the nineteenth century caused Westphalian governance on public health to change dramatically. In response to a series of damaging cholera outbreaks in the first half of the nineteenth century, states, led by the European great powers, began in 1851 to develop systemic diplomatic processes and international legal rules in order to facilitate cooperation on infectious diseases. Over the course of the next century, states constructed a specific governance regime to address the growing problem of cross-border microbial traffic.

The governance regime crafted during this period conformed to the structure and principles of the Westphalian system. The international sanitary conventions negotiated by states in this period (see Table 3.1) reflected, for example, a horizontal governance approach to the international spread of infectious diseases. States were the units of governance, and the rules created sought to mitigate the frictions infectious

Table 3.1 Major International Sanitary Conventions negotiated and/or adopted, 1851–1951

Year	*Convention negotiated and/or adopted*
1851	International Sanitary Conference in Paris negotiated a Convention and Regulations on maritime traffic and control of plague, cholera, and yellow fever. Neither entered into force.
1859	International Sanitary Conference in Paris negotiated a Convention simplifying the 1851 Convention and Regulations. It never entered into force.
1874	International Sanitary Conference in Vienna negotiated a Convention to establish a permanent International Commission on Epidemics. It never entered into force.
1881	International Sanitary Conference in Washington, D.C. negotiated a Convention to establish a permanent International Sanitary Agency of Notification. It never entered into force.
1892	International Sanitary Conference in Venice adopted the International Sanitary Convention of 1892, which entered into force.
1893	International Sanitary Conference in Dresden adopted the International Sanitary Convention of 1893, which entered into force.
1894	International Sanitary Conference in Paris adopted the International Sanitary Convention of 1894, which entered into force.
1897	International Sanitary Conference in Venice adopted the International Sanitary Convention of 1897, which entered into force.
1903	International Sanitary Conference in Paris adopted the International Sanitary Convention of 1903, which replaced the International Sanitary Conventions of 1892, 1893, 1894, and 1897.
1912	International Sanitary Conference in Paris adopted the International Sanitary Convention of 1912, which entered into force.
1926	International Sanitary Conference in Paris adopted the International Sanitary Convention of 1926, which entered into force.
1933	International Sanitary Convention for Aerial Navigation adopted, which entered into force.
1951	World Health Organization adopted the International Sanitary Regulations.

Source: Fidler 1999, pp. 22–3

diseases caused for state interactions, primarily trade and travel. Historians of these efforts stress that a driving force behind the development of an international governance framework for infectious diseases was the increasing drag that national quarantine measures were creating for international trade. Norman Howard-Jones (1975, p. 11) stated that quarantine in the nineteenth century 'resulted in onerous delays and expenditure occasioned by the immobilization of ships, the incarceration of their crews and passengers in lazarets, and the destruction or spoilage of their cargoes.' The burdens of national quarantine measures rose as the speed and volume of international trade increased during the nineteenth century. The rising commercial costs imposed by a system of uncoordinated, unregulated national quarantine practices meant that trade rather than health drove the development of international governance on infectious diseases. As Howard-Jones (1975, p. 11) observed, 'the first faltering steps towards international health cooperation followed trade.' In order to reduce growing frictions in state interactions produced by the convergence of national quarantine measures and growing levels of international trade, the exercise of public health sovereignty by states would need to be regulated.

Under principles of Westphalian governance, the regulation of sovereignty comes from states agreeing to limit their sovereignty through rules of international law. As Table 3.1 indicates, the period from 1851 to 1951 proved fertile for the process of making international law on infectious diseases as states concluded many treaties on infectious disease control. These agreements represented Westphalian governance attempts to balance national public health actions on infectious diseases, such as quarantine, with the desire for an efficient flow in international trade. In this sense, the problem of the cross-border transmission of infectious diseases was slotted directly into the structure and principles of Westphalian governance.

The development of international governance on infectious diseases also reflected the non-intervention principle of the Westphalian system. The regime's focus was on the management of state interactions – trade and travel – not on the public health conditions and problems that existed within the sovereign territories of states. The rules did not penetrate the state to require improvements with respect to national infectious disease control. How a state organized and implemented public health in its own territory was not the subject of infectious disease diplomacy or international law on infectious disease control.

This non-interventionary approach held even when governments knew that the trade frictions created by germs could be mitigated by reducing infectious disease problems *before* the pathogens spread to other countries. For example, the international regimes for infectious disease control crafted in the last half of the nineteenth century and the first half of the twentieth century never required states to improve national sanitation and water systems despite knowledge that such improvements would decrease cholera outbreaks and thus their cross-border spread. The famous nineteenth-century German epidemiologist, Robert Koch, expressed his frustration at the diplomatic activity on infectious disease control by calling the international sanitary conventions 'quite superfluous' and arguing that the international spread of cholera would be stopped if each state seized cholera by the throat and stamped it out (Howard-Jones, 1975, p. 76).

International health organizations created during the first century of international health diplomacy (see Table 3.2) did work with member states to improve national public health capabilities. For example, the Health Organization of the League of Nations (1931, p. 30) noted the following in 1931:

> The public health authorities of all countries benefit from the work of the Epidemiological Service of the Health Organisation and from the experience of its technical committees; they can also at any time request the Health Organisation to place experts at their disposal to carry out specific tasks, and they have in fact done so. Sometimes an opinion is required on measures to cope with malaria, syphilis or an epidemic of dengue, and sometimes the request is for advice on the re-organisation of the public health administration of a whole country.

In the Westphalian system, the provision of such assistance by international health organizations depended entirely on the discretion of the sovereign state, which could ask for, or accept, assistance with national

Table 3.2 International health organizations created between 1851 and 1951

Year	*International health organization*
1902	Pan American Sanitary Bureau
1907	Office International d'Hygiène Publique
1923	Health Organization of the League of Nations
1948	World Health Organization

Source: Fidler 1999, pp. 22–3

public health problems in the exercise of its supreme authority over its territory and people. Westphalian governance included no mandates for a sovereign state to organize its internal infectious disease control policies and programs in specific ways. As the quote from the Health Organization of the League of Nations suggests, sovereign states often did seek assistance with internal public health matters. Sufficient political and especially economic incentives existed for states to be concerned about their territories being the source of cross-border microbial traffic that international health organizations could, and did, play useful roles in Westphalian public health.

Finally, Westphalian public health bore the imprint of the great powers of the international system. The great powers of Europe began to construct a governance regime for infectious diseases in the latter half of the nineteenth century for two basic reasons. First, the European great powers felt vulnerable to the importation of infectious diseases from non-European regions, what were called the 'Asiatic diseases.' As played out in the development of international health diplomacy, fear of disease importation was 'not a wish for the general betterment of the health of the world, but the desire to protect certain favoured (especially European) nations from contamination by their less-favoured (especially Eastern) fellows' (Howard-Jones, 1950, p. 1035).

Second, as mentioned previously, the great powers' interest in facilitating increased flow of international trade created growing impatience with the trade burdens imposed by the decentralized system of national quarantine practices. Goodman (1971, p. 389) noted that '[f]ear of the spread of cholera and, later, plague and yellow fever, together with the obvious economies to trade in a uniform system of quarantine were the two motivations in international health for seventy years or so.' At the forefront of this frustration was the nineteenth century's most powerful state, Great Britain. Britain's extensive empire and global trading interests gave it a particularly strong desire to see international governance develop on infectious disease control in a manner acceptable to British economic interests.

The imprint of the great powers can also be seen in the infectious diseases selected for inclusion in the governance regime. Throughout its history, the international legal rules on infectious disease control addressed only infectious diseases for which trade and travel were considered vectors, such as plague, cholera, and yellow fever. Westphalian public health targeted germ threats considered external to Europe, hence the emphasis on 'Asiatic diseases' seen in the development of international governance on infectious diseases. Infectious diseases endemic to Europe, such as smallpox and tuberculosis, generally did not fall within Westphalian governance for public health despite their cross-border transmissibility. Governance of such endemic diseases remained a matter of the unfettered exercise of sovereignty.

Westphalian public health in action: The International Health Regulations

To make the conceptual overview of Westphalian public health more concrete, this section analyzes the International Health Regulations (IHR) promulgated by the World Health Organization (WHO). The structure, principles, and politics of Westphalian public health governance all appear in the IHR. The IHR also represent the 'classical regime' for international governance on infectious diseases because the IHR are the direct progeny of the approach to infectious disease cooperation developed since the mid-nineteenth century (Fidler, 2003a, pp. 285–6).

Currently, the IHR are the only set of international legal rules binding on WHO member states concerning the control of infectious diseases (WHO, 2002a, p. 63). The IHR formally began life in 1951 as the International Sanitary Regulations (WHO, 2002d, p. 2). WHO adopted the International Sanitary Regulations in 1951 in an effort to consolidate the patchwork of international sanitary conventions in effect prior to World War II into one set of universally applicable rules (Fidler, 1999, p. 59). This consolidation and harmonization effort did not involve moving the regime away from its basic substantive structure, which means that the governance approach developed before WHO's creation formed the basis for the International Sanitary Regulations. WHO changed the name from the International Sanitary Regulations to the IHR in the late 1960s (WHO, 2002d, p. 2), but this name change did not alter the fundamental continuity of the classical regime on infectious disease control. The IHR descend, therefore, directly from the very origins of Westphalian public health governance.

The form the IHR take is in keeping with the Westphalian template. The IHR are binding rules of international law created by WHO member states. Although these rules are called 'regulations,' this moniker does not affect their status as a treaty under international law (Vienna Convention on the Law of Treaties, 1969, Article 2.1(a)). The process through which WHO member states adopted the IHR differs from the normal process of concluding treaties. The IHR were adopted under Articles 21 and 22 of the WHO Constitution (WHO, 1948), under which the World Health Assembly (composed of all WHO member states) can adopt regulations that become binding on a WHO member state unless such state expressly refuses to be bound by the regulations.

Under normal procedures for making treaties, states are not bound unless they expressly agree to be bound by treaties. International lawyers sometimes refer to the normal treaty process as one in which states can 'opt in' and accept a treaty's rules. The process created by the WHO Constitution is, however, an 'opt out' approach because a WHO member state has to declare its intention not to be bound. The WHO Constitution declares in Article 22 that '[r]egulations adopted pursuant to Article 21 shall come into force for all Members after due notice has been given of their adoption by the Health Assembly except for such Members as may notify the Director-General of rejection or reservations within the period stated in the notice.' The 'opt out' approach is merely a procedural device because, at the end of the day, the sovereign state decides whether it will be bound by the rules adopted under Article 21 of the WHO Constitution. The 'opt out' approach is just as Westphalian in this regard as the 'opt in' treaty process.

The substance of the IHR represents classical Westphalian public health governance. The IHR's objective is to ensure the maximum security against the international spread of disease with minimal interference with world traffic (IHR, 1969, Foreword). This objective reflects horizontal governance because it focuses on infectious diseases moving between states. The IHR do not address aspects of public health governance that touch on how a government prevents and controls infectious diseases within its sovereign territory. The limited governance scope of the IHR is also clear from the small number of diseases subject to its rules, currently only plague, cholera, and yellow fever (IHR, 1969, Article 1). In all these respects, the IHR comply with the principle of non-intervention by addressing only aspects of infectious disease control that relate to the intercourse among states.

The IHR's rules for achieving maximum security against the international spread of disease with minimal interference with world traffic also reflect Westphalian tenets of governance. The IHR seek to achieve maximum security against the international spread of disease through two sets of rules. First, the IHR require that WHO member states notify WHO of outbreaks of diseases subject to the Regulations (IHR, 1969, Articles 2–13). This notification requirement serves as the backbone of WHO's international surveillance activities on the diseases subject to the IHR. Surveillance is a critical public health tool for addressing infectious diseases (Institute of Medicine, 1992, p. 2; US CDC, 1994, p. 12).

Surveillance allows public health authorities to know what diseases are circulating in a population and what interventions would be most appropriate. Surveillance on the diseases subject to the IHR provides WHO member states with information that allows them to take rational public health decisions about their travel and trade with the disease-affected nations.

The second category of rules in the IHR that connect to the maximum security against international disease spread involves provisions that require WHO member states to maintain certain public health capabilities at ports and airports (IHR, 1969, Articles 14–22). Ports and airports are the gateways of Westphalian state interaction through trade and travel. To mitigate the possibility of cross-border disease spread, these gateways should not themselves be vectors of microbial traffic by harboring, for examples, rats or mosquitoes that can travel to other countries in planes and ships and spread disease. The IHR's focus on ports and airports contrasts with the absence of any other rules on national public health capabilities, which again is consistent with the principles of sovereignty and non-intervention.

The IHR seek to achieve minimum interference with world traffic by regulating the trade and travel restrictions WHO member states can take against countries suffering outbreaks subject to the Regulations. The IHR provide that the trade and travel measures prescribed for each disease subject to the Regulations are the most restrictive measures that WHO member states may take (IHR, 1969, Article 23). The IHR contain the maximum measures that a WHO member state may apply to address potential cross-border transmissions of cholera, plague, or yellow fever (IHR, 1969, Articles 23–29). The IHR have provisions that prevent the departure of infected persons by means of transportation and that limit actions taken against ships and aircraft en route between ports of departure and arrival, against persons and means of transport upon arrival, and against cargo, goods, baggage, and mail moving in international transport (IHR, 1969, Articles 30–49).

These IHR rules are designed to ensure that infectious disease control measures applied against foreign trade and travel conform to public health principles and scientific evidence. The aim is to reduce public health restrictions on trade and travel to only those that are justifiable on public health grounds. This reason explains why the IHR contain specific provisions that relate to each disease subject to the Regulations and that prescribe, for example, the incubation periods of the diseases (IHR, 1969, Articles 50, 61, and 65). This aspect of the IHR connects to the long-standing goal of Westphalian public health governance to reduce frictions between the exercise of public health sovereignty and the flow of international trade and travel.

The collapse of the classical regime

The IHR represent, and have since their creation in 1951 represented, the classical regime of Westphalian public health governance. The IHR constitute, however, a significant failure for Westphalian public health. This failure extends beyond routine violations of the IHR to touch upon underlying problems with the Westphalian template for infectious disease control. This section analyzes the collapse of the classical regime and its implications for the traditional Westphalian framework for public health.

The IHR failed comprehensively to achieve their objective of maximum security against international disease spread with minimum interference with world traffic. WHO member states routinely violated their IHR obligations to report outbreaks of diseases subject to the Regulations (Dorolle, 1969, p. 104; Delon, 1975, p. 24; CISET, 1995, p. 4; Garrett, 1996, p. 74). A leading reason given for the massive non-compliance with notification duties was that WHO member states did not report outbreaks out of fear of the economic costs they would suffer when countries learned of and reacted to the outbreaks (Dorolle, 1969, pp. 104–5; Delon, 1975, p. 24; CISET, 1995, p. 4; Fidler *et al.*, 1997, p. 778).

This reason for non-compliance would be unpersuasive as long as WHO member states complied with the IHR's rules on trade and travel measures. Unfortunately for the classical regime, non-compliance with these IHR provisions was also epidemic. In 1968, for example, WHO's Deputy Director-General asserted that the objective of avoiding 'excessive and unnecessary quarantine measures' had failed (Dorolle, 1969, p. 105). A 1975 WHO guide to the IHR concluded that '[i]nstances of excessive and useless measures have been numerous in the history of the application of the Regulations since 1951' (Delon, 1975, p. 24).

In essence, the classical regime imploded as WHO member states ignored their international legal obligations under the IHR. In 1969 the WHO Deputy Director-General pronounced the IHR's legal duties on both notification and maximum permissible measures to be a 'dead letter' (Dorolle, 1969, p. 105). Boris Velimirovic (1976, p. 481) asked in frustration whether there was 'much sense in the maintenance of rules if they are not observed – if they are disregarded or more or less systematically broken – without any consequences for those who deviate.'

The classical regime's collapse goes beyond this implosion of non-compliance. In a number of contexts, the IHR simply became irrelevant to infectious disease control. The IHR's focus on what were called 'the pestilential diseases of the past' (Roelsgaard, 1974, p. 267) increasingly made the classical regime irrelevant to more pressing global infectious disease problems. As a governance matter, the IHR were irrelevant to attempts to address diseases not subject to the Regulations.

The significance of the IHR's governance irrelevance became painfully clear in the 1980s. After WHO successfully eradicated smallpox in the late 1970s, in 1981 WHO revised the IHR to remove smallpox from the diseases subject to the Regulations, leaving the current list of cholera, plague, and yellow fever. When HIV/AIDS emerged as a global epidemic in the 1980s, the IHR had no application at all because HIV/AIDS was not a disease subject to the Regulations. Further, WHO never added HIV/AIDS to the IHR's list of diseases because, in part, experts concluded that the IHR's irrelevance could not be fixed by simply adding more diseases to its list (Vignes, 1989). The IHR suffered from deeper flaws.

Some efforts were made to apply the IHR to the HIV/AIDS epidemic in the mid-1980s. As the HIV/AIDS problem became more widely known, a number of countries began to require 'AIDS-free certificates' from international travelers. Some WHO member states asserted that such requirements violated Article 81 of the IHR, which provides that '[n]o health document, other than those provided for in the Regulations, shall be required in international traffic.' With respect to this issue, WHO (1985) asserted that 'no country bound by the Regulations may refuse entry into its territory to a person who fails to provide a medical certificate stating that he or she is not carrying the AIDS virus.' WHO (1986) claimed that 'to require such certificates, let alone to insist on blood tests on arrival, would be totally contrary to the International Health Regulations.'

WHO's legal interpretation of Article 81 of the IHR in connection with 'AIDS-free certificates' was dubious at best given that HIV/AIDS was not a disease subject to the Regulations. Under principles of treaty interpretation, Article 81 cannot be interpreted without reference to Article 23, which contains the general principle on the health measures allowed under the IHR. Requirements for health documents are simply a sub-set of health measures governed by Article 23. Article 23 provides: 'The health measures permitted by these Regulations are the maximum measures applicable to international traffic, which a State may require for the protection of its territory *against the diseases subject to the Regulations*' (emphasis added).

The WHO's interpretation of Article 81 essentially meant any new public health measure – even one justified by public health principles – implemented by a WHO member state to address a threat from a new disease not subject to the IHR was illegal because the measure was not expressly provided for by the Regulations. Even if WHO's legal interpretation of Article 81 had merit at the time, WHO member states continued to ignore it and require 'AIDS-free certificates' and, according to Katarina Tomasevski (1995, p. 868), 'no action has been undertaken to identify instances of noncompliance, or to promote compliance with the sole binding international instrument WHO has produced.' This episode merely underscores the IHR's irrelevance to the HIV/AIDS pandemic.

The IHR also became increasingly irrelevant to the way in which WHO's work on infectious diseases had developed since its creation. Dyna Arhin-Tenkorang and Pedro Conceição (2003, pp. 485–7) trace international health cooperation's move away from 'at the border' controls to 'meeting diseases at their sources.' After its formation in 1948, '[i]n a period of great vitality in the scientific understanding of infectious diseases and of progress in medical technology – in vaccines for prevention and drugs for treatment – the WHO added eliminating communicable diseases at their sources to its mandate of containing their spread through its more traditional functions of coordinating international health regulations and serving as an information clearinghouse' (Arhin-Tenkorang and Conceição, 2003, p. 487).

WHO's desire to attack infectious diseases at their sources within countries represented a vertical public health strategy rather than a horizontal one. Vertical strategies seek to reduce infectious disease prevalence within states (see Figure 3.2).

Vertical strategies are not primarily interested in cross-border microbial traffic, which is the *raison d'être* of the classical regime on infectious

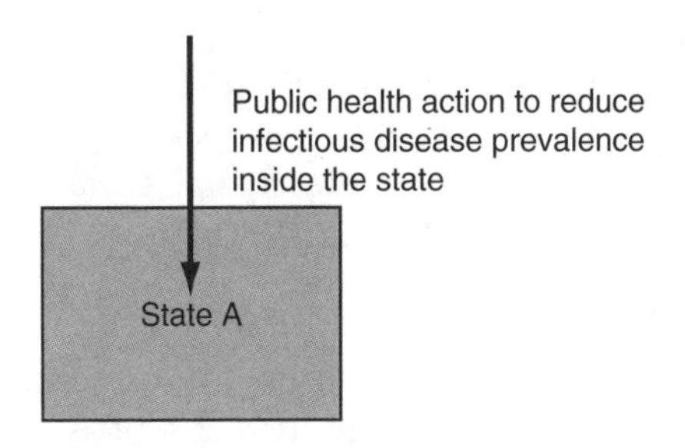

Figure 3.2 Vertical public health strategies

disease control. Reducing infectious disease prevalence inside countries would help reduce cross-border microbial traffic as the likelihood of disease exportation is reduced. The vertical strategy is essentially what Robert Koch advocated when he criticized the international sanitary conventions as superfluous and urged nations to control and eliminate epidemic diseases inside their own borders.

WHO's growing interest in vertical as opposed to horizontal public health strategies extended beyond its activities on eradicating diseases at their sources. WHO's main strategic focus during its 50-plus years has been trying to improve public health in developing countries. Pannenborg (1979, p. 343) described this focus as WHO discarding 'in all its principal policies both the first and the second world[,] almost completely focusing on the LDC-world and enhancing the latter to a special subject of international law.' The IHR were irrelevant to this mission, as was the general Westphalian framework providing the IHR's architecture.

WHO's work with developing countries predominantly involved vertical public health strategies because WHO was more interested in improving public health conditions within poor countries than in managing the public health consequences of mechanistic state interaction for the primary benefit of the great powers. As Arhin-Tenkorang and Conceição (2003, p. 487) argued, '[a]ddressing diseases at their sources required a new type of interaction between governments and WHO. National health authorities provide most of the control of diseases at their sources. But for developing countries without the capacity or resources to control communicable diseases, the WHO helped to do so – funded by industrial countries.' In this shift, humanitarianism replaced the fear and economic concerns of the great powers as the driving force of international health activities.

This shift from horizontal to vertical strategies was also apparent in the increasing role human rights played in public health. The WHO Constitution is the first international legal instrument to state that the right to the highest attainable standard of physical and mental health was a fundamental human right (WHO, 1948, Preamble). The human right to health is radically counter-Westphalian because it makes the individual rather than the state the central governance focus. John Vincent (1986, p. 129) captured the friction between Westphalian politics and human rights when he observed:

> The society of states should and does concern itself with rights, but they are not the rights of individuals, or even nations, but of states. And one of the points about rights recognized by the society

> of states . . . was to allow political diversity, plural conceptions of rights that were to apply to individuals and groups within states. The promotion of human rights, from the point of view of the morality of states, turns this doctrine inside out.

As Vincent's argument pinpoints, the concept of human rights creates immediate tensions with the Westphalian governance principle of non-intervention because the concept invites scrutiny of how a government acts within its territory toward people subject to its sovereignty.

Comparing the Westphalian governance approach in the IHR with WHO's Health for All effort illustrates how Westphalian public health was falling out of favor by the end of the 1970s. The IHR contain no reference to the human right to health, and this right plays no role at all in the mechanics of the Regulations. By the mid-1970s, the horizontal governance failure of the IHR was apparent. The shift in WHO's priorities from horizontal to vertical governance is clear in the Health for All effort. The Health for All initiative sought to make primary health care universally accessible inside every country, which reflects a vertical public health strategy not tied to mechanistic interactions between states.

The language and contents of the Declaration of Alma Ata (1978), which launched the Health for All movement, could not be farther from what appears in the IHR. The Declaration begins with a reaffirmation of health as a fundamental human right, stresses the unacceptability of the inequality in health status of people living in developed and developing countries, connects health promotion to the economic and social objectives of the New International Economic Order, emphasizes the duty of governments to provide adequate health care for all their respective peoples, and focuses on the promotion of primary health care as the means for global health progress. The model of public health governance expressed in the Declaration of Alma Ata is not from the world Westphalia made.

The HIV/AIDS pandemic further highlights the conceptual and policy shifts taking place in public health governance. In trying to address HIV/AIDS, public health experts did not try to retrofit the IHR's Westphalian framework but rather turned to international human rights law to provide governance norms for the fight against this new plague. As Jonathan Mann (1999, p. 217) noted, WHO's emphasis in the latter half of the 1980s on stopping discrimination against those infected with HIV/AIDS represented 'the first time in history [that] preventing discrimination toward those affected by an epidemic became an integral part of a global strategy to prevent and control an epidemic of infectious disease.' Mann and others supported the convergence of public health and human rights, asserting that '[t]he modern movement of human rights . . . provides AIDS prevention with a coherent conceptual framework for identifying and analyzing the societal root causes of vulnerability to HIV' (Mann, 1999, p. 222). Bringing international human rights law to bear on public health meant piercing the sovereign veil and scrutinizing how governments treated their citizens and their health – strategies not supported by Westphalian principles.

The emphasis on human rights in the HIV/AIDS pandemic also stimulated a growing role for non-state actors in public health governance. The human rights strategy made individuals actors in public health governance and brought non-governmental organizations (NGOs) into public health in new ways. NGOs had long played important roles in public health, especially in scientific research and delivering health care services in less affluent countries. NGO activism on health emerged more controversially in the tumultuous 1970s, as illustrated by the campaign by a coalition of NGOs against the marketing of breast-milk substitutes in developing countries by multinational corporations (Loughlin and Berridge, 2002, p. 16). The human rights–public health linkage that developed in connection with HIV/AIDS in the 1980s and 1990s brought new NGOs into public health governance issues, reinforcing the general shift underway from horizontal to vertical strategies.

A final context in which the irrelevance of the Westphalian IHR was apparent concerned the great powers. As discussed earlier, the great powers were the driving force behind the development of the classical regime. Over the course of the twentieth century, the classical regime became increasingly unimportant to the great powers. Most of the great powers succeeded in reducing infectious disease morbidity and mortality in their territories through domestic public health reforms and harnessing the potential of antibiotics and vaccines. The classical regime was irrelevant to the great powers' infectious disease achievements in the twentieth century because such achievements 'do not seem to have needed or relied much, if at all, on international treaties creating international health organizations and regimes on communicable disease control' (Fidler, 2002, p. 45).

Germs still did not recognize the borders of the great powers, but the great powers had created material public health capabilities that allowed them seemingly to cope with the increasing speed and volume of trade and travel and its implications for infectious disease spread. The need of the great powers for the kind of international cooperation embodied in the IHR had all but vanished, leaving the regime without its traditional political engine.

As indicated earlier, the role of the great powers shifted from one of direct concern with the classical regime to one of providing funds to facilitate improvements in public health in developing countries. The politics produced by this shift reflected not only the conflict between democracy and communism but also the growing voice and demands of the developing world, epitomized by the proclamation of a New International Economic Order in 1974. As Kelly Loughlin and Virginia Berridge (2002, p. 16) observed, 'North/South (donor/recipient of aid) became a new axis of political and ideological conflict in postwar international health.'

From Westphalian public health towards what?

The IHR's effective abandonment by the great powers, WHO member states, and WHO itself left the classical regime of Westphalian public health in a governance twilight zone. By the 1990s, the Westphalian model of infectious disease control appeared to be in serious trouble. The classical regime was a failure and, perhaps worse, an irrelevant failure. As the phenomenon of 'emerging and re-emerging infectious diseases' gathered more attention in the early 1990s, the world seemed poised to leave the Westphalian framework behind for something else. The nature of this new governance paradigm was not exactly clear. Developments in the 1970s and 1980s suggested that vertical public health strategies supported by international human rights law and influenced by NGOs would characterize the next generation of governance on infectious disease control. The next chapter continues the tale by analyzing the evolution of new governance concepts for infectious diseases in the 1990s and early 2000s.

4

Public Health in the Post-Westphalian System of Global Politics

Microbes on the march

The decade of the 1990s witnessed a renaissance of interest in infectious diseases in both the public health and political worlds. By the early 1990s, public health experts were growing increasingly concerned about a resurgence of infectious diseases around the world. In 1992, the Institute of Medicine's Committee on Emerging Microbial Threats to Health published its seminal report *Emerging Infections: Microbial Threats to Health in the United States* (Institute of Medicine, 1992). This report marked the beginning of extensive public health and political efforts in the 1990s to come to grips with 'emerging and re-emerging infectious diseases' (EIDs).

The US Centers for Disease Control and Prevention (CDC) defined EIDs as 'diseases of infectious origin whose incidence in humans has increased within the past two decades or threatens to increase in the near future' (US CDC, 1994, p. 1). This definition encompasses not only diseases never previously identified (e.g., HIV/AIDS) but also diseases that many believed had been conquered (e.g., tuberculosis). The inclusion of re-emerging infectious diseases was significant because it focused attention, in many instances, on factors beyond the microbial agent causing the disease. The re-emergence of yellow fever as a public health threat had nothing to do with mutations in the yellow fever virus but was attributable to the breakdown in public health measures, such as mosquito control and widespread vaccination, and to socio-economic changes accelerated by globalization, such as increased urbanization in tropical regions and increased air travel (Institute of Medicine, 1992, p. 40).

From the beginning, analyses of EIDs were sensitive to economic, social, and environmental factors that encouraged the emergence or re-emergence of infectious diseases. For example, the 1992 report from Institute of Medicine's Committee on Emerging Microbial Threats to Health looked beyond the pathogenic agents involved in EIDs and focused on six factors that played a role in emergence and re-emergence: (1) human demographics and behavior; (2) technology and industry; (3) economic development and land use; (4) international travel and commerce; (5) microbial adaptation and change; and (6) breakdown of public health measures (Institute of Medicine, 1992, p. 47). Policy responses to EIDs could not, therefore, concentrate merely on developing new or better antimicrobial technologies.

The size of the EID phenomenon was sufficient, on its own, to catch people's attention. In its 1992 report, the Institute of Medicine's Committee on Emerging Microbial Threats identified 54 emerging and re-emerging infectious agents (Institute of Medicine, 1992, pp. 36–41). In 1995, a US interagency working group identified 29 new infectious diseases and 20 re-emerging diseases since 1973 (CISET, 1995). Although these two studies focused on the EID threat from the perspective of the United States, the literature from this time period also clearly describes the threat in global terms. In fact, the World Health Organization's *World Health Report* for 1996 focused on the infectious disease resurgence and declared that infectious diseases represented a world crisis (WHO, 1996).

EIDs played a prominent role in stimulating analysis in the 1990s on the 'globalization of public health.' This phrase had different meanings and connotations for different analysts, but the basic idea uniting commentators on this topic was the breakdown between the traditional categories of 'national' and 'international' health. In many respects, the novelty of the globalization of public health was exaggerated because, as previous chapters noted, the phenomenon of germs not recognizing borders is quite old. Further, the rise of infectious diseases as a matter of international diplomatic concern in the nineteenth century is attributable to the forces identified in the 1990s literature on the globalization of public health: increased volumes and speed of travel and trade spreading infectious diseases into countries with inadequate or non-existent public health systems. Infectious disease emergence as a byproduct of the processes of globalization was not new.

Another feature of the EID phenomenon in the 1990s echoed what happened when infectious diseases first became a topic of international diplomacy in the mid-nineteenth century. As indicated in Chapter 3, infectious disease control emerged onto the agenda of international politics in the nineteenth century because powerful European states were growing concerned about the importation of 'Asiatic' diseases and the burdens national quarantine measures were imposing on their international trade. International health diplomacy did not have its origins in humanitarian concerns about health conditions in poor, non-European countries. Interestingly, features of the rise of the EID issue in the 1990s exhibit similar characteristics.

Much of the early and most prominent literature on the subject came from the United States, the leading great power in the international system. Following the Institute of Medicine's groundbreaking 1992 report on microbial threats to health in the United States, elements of the US government began to examine and formulate policy for addressing the threat infectious diseases posed to the United States. In 1994, CDC issued its first EID report, *Emerging Infectious Disease Threats: A Prevention Strategy for the United States* (US CDC, 1994). In 1995, an interagency US government working group released *Infectious Disease – A Global Health Threat*, which examined the dangers that the resurgence of infectious diseases posed to US foreign policy and national security interests (CISET, 1995).

The Clinton administration elevated EIDs as a matter of US national and foreign policy in 1996 when Vice President Gore announced a new national initiative to combat EIDs, asserting that 'there is no more menacing threat to our global health today than emerging infectious diseases' (Gore, 1996). US Health and Human Services Secretary Donna Shalala even described the Clinton administration as making war on infectious diseases (McClesky, 1996). As part of this effort, the United States began to include the threat of EIDs on bilateral and multilateral diplomatic agendas, such as bilateral initiatives with Russia and South Africa, G7 summit meetings, and the Asia Pacific Economic Cooperation forum (Fidler, 1997b, pp. 784–5).

These activities, plus others that followed, indicated that infectious diseases had once again become a foreign policy concern of the great powers. The engagement of the United States on this issue in the 1990s helped solidify a diplomatic foothold for the EID issue in a manner that would not have been possible without the backing of the world's remaining superpower. The renaissance of interest in infectious diseases in the 1990s and early 2000s owes much to the threats felt by the United States and the responses this great power began to make. The nineteenth-century emergence of infectious diseases as a matter of international politics occurred for the same reason – the great powers were concerned and willing to exercise their power to reduce the external threat they perceived from infectious diseases.

The influence of great-power concerns can be seen even in the phrase 'emerging and re-emerging infectious diseases.' For many parts of the developing world, infectious diseases had never disappeared as a source of morbidity and mortality. In the developing world, infectious diseases had not un-emerged. As Paul Farmer (1999, p. 39) asked, 'If certain populations have long been afflicted by these disorders, why are the diseases considered "new" or "emerging"? Is it simply because they have come to affect more visible – read, more "valuable" persons?' The use of the term 'emerging and re-emerging infectious diseases' reflects the driving force behind the renaissance in interest in infectious diseases – the powerful once again felt threatened.

These observations on the parallels between the rise of infectious diseases in international politics in the nineteenth century and the return of infectious diseases to diplomatic prominence in the 1990s and early 2000s do not imply that all was the same. The globalization of public health in the late twentieth century had characteristics not seen in the last half of the nineteenth century. The speed of travel and trade had, for example, increased exponentially as transportation technologies, especially jet aircraft, advanced. As EID literature often pointed out, the speed of modern transportation means that a traveler could carry a pathogenic microbe anywhere in the world within twenty-four hours and seed an outbreak.

The volume of trade and travel had also increased enormously since the nineteenth century. Trade liberalization regimes, such as the General Agreement on Tariffs and Trade (GATT, 1947), helped increase the trade in food and food products significantly. The number of people crossing international borders each year for business, tourism, or to escape tyranny, persecution, war, and poverty was also far greater in the late twentieth than the late nineteenth century.

Finally, travel and trade in the late twentieth century were far more global than their precursors a century before. The great powers of the nineteenth century had global trading networks and interests in many regions of the world. Although the sun never set on the British empire, the global nature of travel and trade today dwarfs that of the nineteenth century. More countries and people are more deeply connected economically and technologically in the contemporary era of globalization than at any other time in history. If not yet representing a global village, advances in transportation and information technologies linked human populations into a globalized society without historical precedent.

With the microbes once again on the march, governance questions loomed large, as they had in the mid-nineteenth century when the globalization of public health first forced states to respond systemically. Chapter 3 explored the nature of the governance response constructed from the mid-nineteenth century onwards and that still, despite its glaring weaknesses and the challenges being mounted by vertical public health strategies linked to human rights, formed the prevailing governance architecture when EIDs burst onto the public health and political scene in the early 1990s. Much of the EID literature contained policy recommendations (e.g., strengthen international cooperation) that, if implemented, would merely retrofit Westphalian public health governance without radically changing its structure, principles, or political dynamics. But the EID crisis also began to stimulate thinking outside the Westphalian box in an effort to construct a governance strategy worthy of the challenge the marching microbes now presented.

The shock of the new: Crafting post-Westphalian public health

Public health was not the only field of endeavor to be affected by the forces of globalization in the 1990s and early 2000s. For example, the study and practice of business, law, medicine, and politics all reacted to the ways globalization was changing landscapes and shifting boundaries. Many experts believed that globalization transformed how we think about time and space, changing from top-to-bottom how problems should be addressed. Many phenomena seemed to join the germs because they, too, did not recognize borders.

While many disciplines struggled with the deterritorialization effect of globalized human relations, public health had long understood the epidemiological gossamer borders represent against the spread of pathogenic microbes. Borders remained, however, very prominent in the traditional governance responses to infectious diseases explored in Chapter 3. Even the movement toward vertical public health strategies in the 1970s reflected traditional boundaries, prompting Charles Pannenborg (1979, p. 343) to argue that 'WHO is at best moving towards a new national health order instead of a new international health order.'

In the new era of the globalization of public health, the governance question for public health was how to manage borderless bugs in a borderless world. The 'shock of the new' for public health was not the borderlessness of germs but the realization that infectious disease control in the new global era required more than simply retrofitting Westphalian public health governance. Although literature on the globalization of public health sounded retrofitting themes, such as infectious disease control requires improved international cooperation, discourse on EIDs in the 1990s and early 2000s cast critical light on the Westphalian approach to public health, indicating that this approach to infectious diseases was bankrupt. This bankruptcy was apparent in connection with the structure, principles, and politics of Westphalian public health.

In terms of structure, the state-centric governance framework of Westphalian public health came under scrutiny. Although the state would remain important in any governance framework, the processes of globalization had rendered a state-centric governance focus questionable. As the collapse of the International Health Regulations demonstrated, states had not proved particularly good stewards of horizontal governance on infectious diseases. The state-centric approach led governance toward principles based on politically impermeable borders not on the nature of the borderless risks states and peoples faced.

The principles of sovereignty, non-intervention, and consent-based international law characterized the substance of Westphalian public health. These principles were not designed with public health in mind; they were designed to provide international politics with an orderly and stable framework. Borders were critical concepts to the Westphalian project because the borders represented the demarcation of sovereignty. When public health arose as a concern for diplomatic activity, infectious disease control, understandably, was simply slotted into the long-standing Westphalian template for international relations. The demise of the classical regime on infectious disease control demonstrated how ill-suited the core Westphalian principles were to effective global infectious disease policy.

Bankruptcy was also apparent in the politics of Westphalian public health. Connecting infectious disease control closely to the interests and influence of the great powers had proved unfortunate for infectious disease control. As the great powers got their public health houses in order, their interest in international infectious disease control (which they had started) waned. Public health transformed from an issue in which the self-interests of the great powers were politically and economically engaged to one which the great powers treated as a mere humanitarian endeavor – a public health version of *noblesse oblige*. The lack of interest in, and complacency about, infectious diseases by the great powers during the second half of the twentieth century helped produce the EID crisis, especially the horrifying growth of the HIV/AIDS pandemic.

Similarly, the construction of the main international regime on infectious disease control, eventually embodied by the International Health

Regulations, to target mainly the infectious disease concerns of the great powers proved myopic and inappropriate given the suffering developing countries experienced from infectious diseases. The classical regime's objective of balancing maximum security against international disease spread with minimum interference with world traffic did not speak to the main infectious disease problems facing developed or developing countries. WHO's movement toward vertical public health strategies and human rights norms, which focused on helping developing countries, illustrated the inappropriateness of basing an infectious disease governance strategy on the International Health Regulations' narrow basis.

Although the case against Westphalian public health governance was powerful, public health faced a policy conundrum: How can infectious disease governance be de-Westphalianized in a political environment still deeply rooted in the Westphalian approach? One could rail against state-centrism and sovereignty, but neither states nor sovereignty were going to disappear as factors to consider in constructing governance strategies. Whatever governance approach eventually taken would have 'to confront somehow a fundamental paradox: globalization jeopardizes disease control nationally by eroding sovereignty, while the need for international solutions allows sovereignty to frustrate disease control internationally' (Fidler, 1996, p. 83). Was there a way out of this conundrum, or was public health facing, like other areas of social endeavor grappling with globalization's impact, the 'tyranny of the actual' (Allott, 1999, p. 49)?

New process, new substance

The EID threat and other globalized public health problems stimulated new thinking in the 1990s and early 2000s, which began to shape strategies on process and substance different from the Westphalian model. This new thinking sought to avoid the dead end Westphalian public health had become and the dead end that radical idealism would become in an international system still rooted in the Westphalian model. On the process side, the concept of 'global health governance' emerged as a framework for governance distinct from the state-centric approach. The global health governance concept developed from both empirical and normative analyses. Experts began to examine the increasing role that non-state actors, such as multinational corporations (MNCs) and non-governmental organizations (NGOs), were playing in national and international public health (Dodgson *et al.*, 2002). Facts on the ground demonstrated that this trend was not academic daydreaming.

Normatively, public health experts began to debate the wisdom of harnessing non-state actor participation in the process of governing public health issues. Richard Dodgson, Kelley Lee, and Nick Drager (2002, p. 19) argued, for example, that 'states and state-defined governance alone is not enough. Forms of governance that bring together more concertedly state and non-state actors will be central in a global era.'

On the substance side, the concept of 'global public goods for health' (GPGH) gained increasing attention. This concept flowed directly from increased academic and policy attention on the production of 'global public goods' (Kaul *et al.*, 1999a). A leading definition of a global public good argued that such a good exhibits five characteristics (Kaul *et al.*, 1999b, pp. 9–11). First, consumption of the good is non-rivalrous, in the sense that one person's consumption of the good does not diminish another person's consumption of it. A classic example of a non-rivalrous public good is a traffic light – one driver's use of the light does not prevent another driver from using the light later (Kaul *et al.*, 1999b, pp. 3–4).

Second, consumption of the good is non-excludable. In other words, the good in question is accessible for all elements of society to consume and is not reserved for one segment of society to utilize (Kaul *et al.*, 1999b, pp. 3–4). The third, fourth, and fifth characteristics of a global public good extend the non-excludability principle on a global scale. Thus, a global public good must be of benefit to (1) more than one group of countries; (2) a broad spectrum of socio-economic groups across nations; and (3) present generations without jeopardizing the needs of future generations (Kaul *et al.*, 1999b, pp. 10–11).

Although the definition of 'global public goods' of Kaul *et al.* is well known, experts have criticized and reformulated their definition. David Woodward and Richard Smith (2003, p. 9) redefine, for example, a global public good to mean 'a good which it is rational, from the perspective of a group of nations collectively, to produce for universal consumption, and for which it is irrational to exclude an individual nation from its consumption, irrespective of whether that nation contributes to its financing.' Woodward and Smith's definition keeps non-rivalrous and non-excludable consumption as part of the substance of a global public good. In addition, their definition also focuses on the need for the public good in question to be accessible by more than one country; or, as Woodward and Smith (2003, p. 8) put it, global public goods have to exhibit 'a significant degree of publicness (i.e., non-excludability and non-rivalry) *across national boundaries*' that involves 'more than two nations, with at least one outside the traditional regional groupings (e.g. Europe, Sub-Saharan Africa, or South East Asia) of the other(s).'

Woodward and Smith (2003, pp. 7–8) reject linking the concept of global public goods to population and generational boundaries.

Reconciling competing definitions of 'global public goods' is beyond the scope of this chapter. The main point is to draw attention to the application of the 'global public good' concept to public health problems. For purposes of my analysis, the idea that certain policy interventions can produce GPGH is central. Interventions that qualify as GPGH produce improvements in health that generate positive global externalities. According to Woodward and Smith (2003, pp. 10–13), policy interventions that produce the prevention or containment of communicable diseases and/or general economic benefits can be categorized as GPGH. But, they stress, only the prevention or containment of certain communicable diseases – those with global scope and significant potential of cross-border transmission and onward transmission (e.g., HIV/AIDS, tuberculosis, antimicrobial resistance) – qualifies as a GPGH (Woodward and Smith, 2003, pp. 11, 24–5).

The following sections elaborate on 'global health governance' and 'global public goods for health' by showing how significantly they differ from the Westphalian approach and exploring how these ideas filtered into thinking about infectious disease control in the era of globalization.

Beyond state-centrism: Global health governance

As discussed in Chapter 3, Westphalian public health is premised on the principle that states constitute the only legitimate actors for governance purposes. The Westphalian moment in the seventeenth century represented the effective abandonment of the legitimacy of transnational, non-state actors, such as the Catholic Church, that had played governance roles in earlier times. The Peace of Westphalia stripped governance of international relations bare of such actors and grounded governance in the interactions of sovereign states.

The state-centrism of the Westphalian approach is visible in international public health regimes. WHO is an intergovernmental organization established by states to facilitate their interactions on public health matters. Dodgson *et al.* (2002, p. 18) emphasized the state-centrism of intergovernmental organizations working on health issues:

> Health-related regional organizations (e.g., PAHO, European Union), along with major international health organizations such as WHO and the World Bank are formally governed by member states. Their mandates, in turn, are defined by their role in supporting national

> health systems of those member states. The universality of their activities is measured by the number of member states participating in them. Defining criteria and measures of progress to address the burden of disease, health determinants and health status are focused on the state or groups of states affected.

The International Health Regulations (IHR) also reflect the state-centric framework, especially with regard to the flow of epidemiological information to and from WHO. Under the IHR, surveillance information that WHO can disseminate to its member states can only come from governments (IHR, 1969, Article 11). As WHO (2002d, p. 3) observed, '[t]he IHR wholly depend on the affected country to make an official notification to WHO once cases are diagnosed.' WHO has no legal authority under the IHR to disclose disease outbreak information it receives from reliable non-governmental sources. In addition to the government-only surveillance system, the IHR's provisions address only states. The IHR require WHO member states to maintain certain public health capabilities at ports and airports and to limit their trade- and travel-restricting health measures to those prescribed in the Regulations (IHR, 1969). Non-state actors are neither participants in nor subjects of the IHR.

The state-centric approach seen in the WHO and the IHR reflect 'international governance' – governance between and among states. In contrast to international health governance, global health governance includes not only states and intergovernmental organizations but also non-state actors, such as NGOs and MNCs, as participants in the governance process (Lee and Dodgson, 2003, p. 138). The distinction made between international and global health governance does not mean that non-state actors have never participated in global health endeavors before the end of the twentieth century. NGOs, such as the Rockefeller Foundation, have played important global public health roles for decades, especially in the areas of research and delivery of health care services.

The WHO Constitution recognized the importance of NGOs to public health when it created a process through which NGOS could establish 'official relations' with WHO (WHO, 1948, Article 71). WHO's collaboration with NGOs has the following objectives: 'to promote the policies, strategies and programmes derived from the decisions of the Organization's governing bodies; to collaborate with regard to various WHO programmes in jointly agreed activities to implement these strategies; and to play an appropriate role in ensuring the harmonizing of intersectoral interests among the various sectoral bodies concerned in a country, regional or global setting' (WHO, 1988, p. 74). WHO's contact with NGOs can be informal or formal, with the only category of formal relations being known as 'official relations' (WHO, 1988, p. 74).

NGOs in official relations with WHO have the following privileges: (1) the right to appoint a representative to participate, without the right to vote and under certain conditions, in WHO's meetings or in those of the committees and conferences convened under WHO authority; and (2) access to non-confidential documentation and such other documentation as the WHO Director-General may make available (WHO, 1988, pp. 78–9).

The WHO process of official relations for NGOs demonstrates that international health governance saw value in having intergovernmental health organizations and their member states collaborate with NGOs in the pursuit of public health objectives. Literature on global health governance does not, however, focus on the type of NGO involvement in public health created by the official relations process. Although this process invites NGOs to provide input on international health governance, state-centrism still impedes NGO involvement. First, the official relations process is designed to have NGO input flow into international health governance. This approach does not alter or challenge the Westphalian conception of governance because states remain the primary, legitimate governance actors.

Second, the official relations process only offers the opportunity to effect change through the existing framework of international health governance. More potent forms of influence may exist for NGOs outside this framework. The power of NGO networks and strategic alliances formed outside the formal participatory mechanisms in United Nations bodies provides the best example why NGOs may prefer to effect change from without rather than from within. Such networks and strategic alliances form a political counterweight to the state-centric dynamic of international health governance. Some well-known efforts of NGO policy activism on public health, such as the International Baby Food Action Network's actions against MNC marketing of breast-milk substitutes in the developing world and *Médecins Sans Frontières's* Campaign for Access to Essential Medicines, owe little, if any, of their success to official relations with WHO. These efforts brought pressure to bear directly on states, international health organizations, and MNCs from the outside.

Analysis of the official relations process also suggests that this approach may have become anachronistic. A 2002 study of NGO official relations with WHO reported that 189 NGOs were in official relations but an additional 240 NGOs not in official relations had informal relations with WHO at its Geneva headquarters (Lanord, 2002, p. 5). Thus, more than 55 per cent of WHO contacts with NGOs take place outside the official relations process (Lanord, 2002, p. 5). In 1948, when the WHO Constitution came into force, official relations for NGOs probably seemed quite a progressive move within the Westphalian template. More than 50 years later, the capabilities of NGOs to network globally, reach policy makers, and influence national and international policy have grown enormously. In short, the majority of NGOs with interests in public health appear to have concluded that the most effective way to influence health policy is not through official relations with WHO.

The official relations process also does not recognize the participation in governance of for-profit, non-state actors, the MNCs. Experts have argued that globalization increases the power of MNCs over national and international policy (Willets, 2001, pp. 362–6), which power MNCs exercise without requiring 'official relations' with international organizations. MNCs have independent power that they can bring to bear on the state-centric machinery of international health governance.

The concept of global health governance focuses on something very different from, and more radical than, WHO's official relations model. Global health governance stands for the proposition that governance of public health issues must include not only state actors but also non-state actors. The radical break with the Westphalian model comes in the belief that non-state actors are legitimate governance actors in their own right. Trying to shoehorn NGO participation into the state-centric framework, as attempted in the official relations process, dilutes what non-state actors bring to the governance table. The elevation of the role of non-state actors in public health governance breaks down the traditional governance borders established by Westphalian principles. To govern an increasingly borderless world requires, in essence, increasingly borderless governance. As Lee and Dodgson (2003, p. 138) argued, '[g]lobal governance views the globe as a single place within which the boundaries of the interstate system and nation-state have been eroded.'

The various roles non-state actors play in global health governance boil down to two categories: antagonist and protagonist roles. In the antagonist role, non-state actors mobilize their members and resources to change the direction of existing public health policy. Antagonist campaigns target an ineffective status quo or challenge new policy initiatives that non-state actors perceive to be insufficient, counterproductive, or regressive.

The previously mentioned International Baby Food Action Network and the Campaign for Access to Essential Medicines provide examples of the antagonist role of non-state actors in health governance. The International Baby Food Action Network launched a global campaign against MNC marketing of breast-milk substitutes in developing countries. This Network proved a successful antagonist as its campaign led eventually to the 1981 adoption by WHO of the International Code of Marketing on Breast-Milk Substitutes (Shubber, 2000). More recently, *Médecins Sans Frontières*'s Campaign for Access to Essential Medicines has had significant impact on global health policy on drug access, perhaps most notably the adoption of the Declaration on TRIPS and Public Health adopted by member states of the World Trade Organization at the Doha Ministerial meeting in November 2001 (WTO, 2001).

Importantly, the antagonist role for non-state actors reflects the shift in governance away from state centrism for two reasons. First, non-state actors playing the antagonist can have independent impact on the making of public health policy by states and intergovernmental organizations. Second, and perhaps more interestingly, the antagonist role is not played exclusively against state actors. Both the campaign against the marketing of breast-milk substitutes and for access to essential medicines witnessed NGOs playing the antagonist against MNCs as well as governments and international organizations.

The International Baby Food Action Network organized a boycott against MNCs marketing breast-milk substitutes in developing countries, and *Médecins Sans Frontières* has criticized pharmaceutical MNCs in its effort to increase access to essential medicines for people in the developing world. NGO efforts directly against MNCs reflect the extent to which NGOs perceive MNCs as non-state actors influencing the direction of public health governance. In response, MNCs have to pick up the gauntlet thrown down by NGOs and battle for their desired policy outcomes. Non-state actors then become joined in a struggle with each other over the substance of health governance in the globalized world. This scenario illustrates why NGOs today may perceive the process of 'official relations' with WHO as a quaint artifact of a bygone age.

The second type of role played by non-state actors in global health governance is the protagonist role. In this role, the non-state actor is not the adversary of the status quo or the opponent of proposed change. Protagonism means that non-state actors are principal players in the creation of new governance policies and interventions. The best example of non-state actor protagonism can be found in the formation of so-called 'public–private partnerships' on global health problems. As the name suggests, these mechanisms are expressly not state-centric because principal contributors come from the private sector, whether for-profit or non-profit. Public–private partnerships have attracted much attention in public health literature in the last few years (Buse and Walt, 2000a; Buse and Walt, 2000b; Widdus, 2001; Buse and Walt, 2002; Reich, 2002). WHO has described the proliferation of public–private partnerships that address infectious diseases as constituting a force that is 'reshaping the landscape of public health' (WHO, 2002a, p. 22).

Two prominent examples of public–private partnerships help clarify the protagonist role non-state actors play in public health governance today. The first example involves the public–private partnership formed between WHO and NGOs in the creation of the Framework Convention for Tobacco Control. Although the intended product of the effort was the classical Westphalian tool of a treaty between states, the process through which the treaty came into being deliberately involved NGO participation at every possible step (Collin, 2003, p. 84). Dodgson *et al.* (2002, p. 20) argued that '[t]hese efforts to build formal links with such a diverse range of stakeholders to support global tobacco control policy is unprecedented for WHO, and a good example of emerging forms of G[lobal] H[ealth] G[overnance].' Anti-tobacco NGOs thus played a protagonist role in bringing the Framework Convention for Tobacco Control into being. Appropriately, the first treaty ever adopted by WHO under Article 19 of its Constitution strongly reflects global health governance through the protagonist participation of NGOs.

The second example concerns the Global Fund to Fight AIDS, Tuberculosis, and Malaria (Global Fund). The 'purpose of the Fund is to attract, manage and disburse additional resources through a new public–private partnership that will make a sustainable and significant contribution to the reduction of infections, illness and death, thereby mitigating the impact caused by HIV/AIDS, tuberculosis and malaria in countries in need, and contributing to poverty reduction' (Global Fund, 2003a). The concept and structure of the Global Fund are about as un-Westphalian as one could imagine. First, the Global Fund is not a classical international organization established by treaty. Its governance structure includes NGOs as voting members (Global Fund, 2003b). Thus, although states play an important role in the Global Fund, states do not monopolize policy because of the formal governance participation of NGOs.

The Global Fund also does not rely on the traditional Westphalian public health reliance on international agreements between states. The Global Fund is not a treaty-based organization, such as WHO, nor an entity embedded in formal intergovernmental structures, such as UNAIDS. The Global Fund is, rather, a non-profit entity established under Swiss law (Global Fund, 2003c). In legal form, the Global Fund looks more like an NGO than an intergovernmental institution. Financial commitments by states to the Global Fund are also not based in treaty law, as are contributions to WHO, because the Fund involves no treaty obligations for states.

Third, the Global Fund is designed to provide financial resources for national-level prevention and treatment projects on HIV/AIDS, tuberculosis, and malaria (Global Fund, 2003a). The Global Fund seeks to implement, thus, vertical public health strategies on infectious disease prevention and control. The vertical approach also distinguishes the Global Fund from the horizontal strategies prevalent in Westphalian public health. The funding approach also makes the Global Fund different from traditional international health organizations, such as WHO, which are not funding agencies for national public health projects. In essence, the Global Fund is designed to redistribute financial resources from rich to poor countries for public health purposes. Although much of the work of WHO and other international health organizations focuses on developing countries, none has had the explicit mandate to redistribute financial resources from rich to poor countries.

Innovation is also present in how the Global Fund carries out its funding mandate. The Global Fund subjects project proposals to scientific and technical scrutiny to ensure that only projects based on scientific evidence and public health principles receive funding (Global Fund, 2003d). The criteria for being funded include the principle that the proposed project involves not only government but also non-governmental participation (Global Fund, 2003d). The public–private partnership dynamic of the Global Fund is, thus, replicated at the level of national projects. Such a requirement is simply not found in the traditional Westphalian public health architecture of international organizations and international law.

The Global Fund's mandate to address the three most serious infectious diseases in the world through vertical public health strategies is also important from the perspective of governance on infectious disease control. States, international organizations, and non-state actors looked at the horrific toll HIV/AIDS, tuberculosis, and malaria were taking on the developing world; and the policy response was not to retrofit the old Westphalian public health architecture again. Instead, global health governance was instituted in the form of a public–private partnership, in which non-state actors play protagonist roles at the global and local levels. The Global Fund's incorporation of non-state actors into its governing architecture and its requirement that funded projects involve civil society participation moves the effort away from international governance toward global governance. Such global governance occurs without the use of Westphalian treaty law or intergovernmental structures.

The Global Fund's support of vertical public health strategies on the prevention and treatment of infectious diseases within developing countries resonates with the movement in public health in the latter half of the twentieth century away from the horizontal approach embedded in the Westphalian system. Other public–private partnerships in the area of infectious diseases have similar vertical ambitions. WHO (2002a, p. 22) notes that public–private partnerships for infectious diseases 'fall into two broad categories: to discover new drugs and vaccines for diseases neglected by research and industry, and to vastly improve access by the poor to existing products.' Absent from these objectives are assuaging the fear and economic concerns of the great powers in connection with trade and travel spreading infectious diseases.

Beyond the national interest: Global public goods for health

The pursuit of global public goods for health (GPGH) represents the second major break from Westphalian public health that developed in the 1990s and early 2000s. As explored earlier, the classical regime on infectious disease control sought to reduce problems cross-border microbial traffic caused. The national interests of states, predominantly the great powers, determined the horizontal nature of the classical regime.

After experiencing successive waves of disease epidemics in the first half of the nineteenth century, the major European powers feared the importation of infectious diseases into their territories. A central objective of the classical regime was to mitigate the national damage imported infectious diseases could cause. The classical regime further served the national interests of the major European powers by creating rules to regulate the application of national quarantine measures in order to reduce the economic costs such measures were increasingly imposing on international trade.

As described earlier, GPGH represent a departure from the narrow, great-power biased objectives of the Westphalian regime on infectious diseases. A GPGH is a product or service connected to the protection or promotion of human health that exhibits a significant degree of non-rivalry and non-excludability in consumption across national boundaries and traditional regional groupings (Woodward and Smith,

2003, p. 8). The GPGH concept deviates from Westphalian public health in terms of producers and consumers.

The producers of the policy outcomes sought under the classical regime on infectious disease control were states, led by the great powers, assisted by intergovernmental organizations. Under Westphalian governance principles, the only possible producers of international legal regimes, such as the IHR, were states. The consumers of the outcomes of the classical regime were likewise states, with the major powers of international politics as prime consumers.

GPGH differ from the Westphalian public health production model because the production process for GPGH involves not only governments and international organizations but also non-state actors, such as NGOs and MNCs. This production process resonates with the ambitions of global health governance to include non-state actors in the process of public health governance. As with global health governance, public–private partnerships provide the best illustrations of the production process innovation in the GPGH concept. For example, public–private partnerships designed to develop new vaccines and drugs for infectious diseases, such as HIV/AIDS, malaria, and tuberculosis, bring together governmental, intergovernmental, and non-governmental resources in attempts to produce technologies designed to improve health globally, but especially in the developing world.

Public–private partnerships could also be used to produce non-tangible goods of global benefit. The public–private partnership between WHO and anti-tobacco NGOs helped create a globally accessible process for fighting the epidemic in tobacco-related diseases. The Framework Convention on Tobacco Control is not the GPGH; the global anti-tobacco process, of which the Framework Convention is part, is the GPGH (Taylor *et al.*, 2003, p. 227). Similarly, the Global Fund creates a GPGH in the process it establishes for the distribution of resources from rich to poor countries in the fight against three terrible disease killers.

One might argue that a 'process' cannot be a public good but could only produce a public good. The jury may still be out on whether the innovative governance processes for global tobacco control and fighting HIV/AIDS, tuberculosis, and malaria produce outcomes that could be called GPGH. This critique has some merit. Some commentators have argued that international regimes, such as the IHR and the Framework Convention on Tobacco Control, are GPGH, or are 'intermediate' GPGH (Kaul, Grunberg, and Stern, 1999, p. 13; Taylor *et al.*, 2003, p. 219) or 'enabling goods' (Giesecke, 2003, p. 209). Formal international agreements themselves are not GPGH, and this conclusion holds whether or not the agreement is successful in achieving its objective. GPGH are predominantly outcomes that result from formal or informal agreements and arrangements.

How, then, can a 'process,' such as the ones used to create the Framework Convention on Tobacco Control and the Global Fund, constitute a GPGH? The answer to this question lies in the fact that sometimes process is substance. In other words, the producers of the process, and the consumers of process' production, value the process itself in addition to its outcome. Take, for example, the commitment of democratic states to the process of democracy. At times, the actual outcomes of the democratic process (e.g., statutes) are abject failures and could not qualify as public goods in any sense. The producers and consumers of democratic governance remain committed to democracy in spite of the shortcomings of what it sometimes produces. The democratic process itself is a public good because it connects with, and expresses, deeply held values about the good society.

The same is true in connection with seeing global governance processes, such as the global tobacco campaign and the Global Fund, as GPGH. The more inclusive, participatory governance processes exhibited in these efforts connect with values about increasing the voice of those affected by globalization in order to promote better prospects for addressing the plight of those most in need on the planet. Great-power dominance of governance does not express contemporary values about the structure and dynamics of the good globalized society. Global governance processes increase the number of stakeholders in policy initiatives, increasing the likelihood that both governmental and non-governmental forces will work together to improve the status quo when the critical stage of implementation is reached.

As for consumers, GPGH conceive of their consumers far more broadly than the traditional Westphalian approach, which fixates on states and their national interests. The definition of a global public good requires that the good exhibit significant non-rivalry and non-excludability in consumption across national boundaries and across traditional regional groupings (Woodward and Smith, 2003, p. 8). The great powers may consume GPGH because these goods are highly non-excludable in terms of consumption; but, unlike the classical regime on infectious diseases, the GPGH concept reaches out to include the weaker elements of globalized society, developing countries and specific disadvantaged populations across borders, as consumers.

This analysis of the GPGH concept does not pretend that this idea is universally accepted or completely coherent in its application. Like any new concept, the term has been the subject of confusion, misapplication, and criticism (Mooney and Dzator, 2003). In some respects, it has become a trendy rhetorical device used by advocates as a way to catch the eye of the media, policy makers, or funding organizations. Smith and Woodward (2003, p. 247) warn that, 'as the GPG concept becomes 'fashionable,' it faces the real possibility of becoming over-exposed, and even abused..., with the natural result that the concept becomes devalued, treated with skepticism and, eventually, with cynicism.' This reality is no reason to dismiss the notion out of hand. After all, many concepts, such as democracy, are subject to controversy in their meaning and misapplication in their implementation.

The rise of the GPGH concept in health policy-making can be glimpsed in the findings of the Commission on Macroeconomics and Health (2001, p. 17), which argued that '[a]n effective assault on diseases of the poor will also require substantial investments in global public goods, including increased collection and analysis of epidemiological data, surveillance of infectious diseases, and research and development into diseases that are concentrated in poor countries (often, though not exclusively, tropical diseases).' The Commission's action agenda included the recommendation (2001, p. 19) that the supply of global public goods, such as international disease surveillance, be bolstered through additional financing of relevant international organizations, including WHO. The Commission (2001, p. 76) captured why the GPGH concept differs from the policy objectives targeted in Westphalian governance when it observed that global public goods 'are public goods that are underprovided by local and national governments, since the benefits accrue beyond a country's borders.' GPGH require thinking about public health outside the Westphalian box of the 'national interest.' In addition, GPGH demand approaches to the collective action problems they pose that go beyond the state-centric framework of the Westphalian template.

Revision of the International Health Regulations: The de-Westphalianization of the classical regime

This chapter has used examples from the area of infectious disease control, such as the Global Fund, to illustrate the public health movement toward global health governance and GPGH. The 1990s and early 2000s also witnessed efforts to embed these governance innovations into the classical regime on infectious disease control, embodied in the IHR. Exploring these efforts provides, thus, an excellent lens to examine the development of post-Westphalian public health in the area of infectious disease control. Prior to the SARS outbreak, the revision of the IHR suffered from obscurity in the ferment of thinking on global health governance and GPGH taking place in the 1990s and early 2000s (Fidler, 2003a, p. 286). This revision process connects, however, to the main concepts evolving in the growing discourse on public health and governance in the age of globalization.

Acknowledging the IHR's failure as a governance mechanism, WHO began in 1995 a process of revising the Regulations to make them more effective in the face of the globalized threat of EIDs (World Health Assembly, 1995; WHO, 1995). As mentioned earlier, the question of revising the IHR during the emergence of HIV/AIDS produced the negative response that merely adding to the list of diseases subject to the Regulations would prove futile. WHO member states would no more comply with disease notification requirements, or maximum prescribed travel-restricting measures, in relation to HIV/AIDS than they had compiled with similar legal duties concerning every other disease made subject to the IHR. In the big picture, the governance problem with the IHR was not the short list of diseases to which they applied. Something more fundamental had to be fixed.

From the beginning of the IHR revision process, WHO decided to keep the IHR's main objective: maximum security against the international spread of disease with minimum interference with world traffic (WHO, 1995). Given the IHR's historical pedigree, WHO's choice to continue the long-standing objective of the classical regime ensured some continuity in this area of public health governance. But, given the IHR's bleak history, this decision seems, at first glance, odd. Would not the perpetuation of this conservative objective doom WHO to repeat the mistakes of the past, and thus perpetuate the failed Westphalian public health governance template? The answer to this question depended on how WHO sought to achieve this traditional objective, and whether the path it selected would transform the objective's meaning into something more radical.

From the earliest stages of the IHR revision process, WHO identified a number of ideas to improve the IHR's contribution to infectious disease governance, and one of the most important, if not the most important, ideas resonates with the global health governance and GPGH concepts – supplement disease reporting by governments with epidemiological information supplied by non-governmental sources. Three conclusions fostered the advancement of this proposal.

First, the proposal connects to the critical importance of surveillance to the control and prevention of infectious diseases. Epidemiological surveillance is 'the systematic collection, analysis and public health response to the occurrence of infectious disease conditions in our communities' and 'encompasses both the reporting and investigation of cases and the submission of clinical specimens when needed for testing at a... public health laboratory' (Emerging Infections Hearings, 1995, pp. 30–1). As one expert put it, '[w]ithout the ability to know with accuracy when, where, and why infectious diseases are occurring, we cannot begin to prevent them' (Emerging Infections Hearings, 1995, p. 31). Surveillance provides baseline information public health officials need to respond to infectious disease threats and to assign priorities to prevention and control efforts concerning different diseases.

Surveillance is, thus, critical to good governance on infectious diseases. Every plan promulgated to improve national and international responses to EIDs in the 1990s and early 2000s makes infectious disease surveillance the most important element in the proposed strategy. The centrality of surveillance to infectious disease governance meant that WHO's revision of the IHR would have to include a surveillance regime that provided adequate and timely data to allow public health responses to be planned and implemented.

The second conclusion that led WHO to the proposal to include non-governmental information in its infectious disease surveillance system was the knowledge that the existing IHR surveillance system had proved grossly inadequate for one fundamental reason – WHO member states routinely failed to comply with their legally binding notification requirements under the IHR. The rather short list of diseases subject to the IHR was another serious problem with the IHR's surveillance system; but, as the IHR revision debates concerning HIV/AIDS suggested, merely adding more diseases was not going to address adequately the problem of non-compliance. The state-centric nature of the IHR's surveillance system was the key problem. Put another way, Westphalian public health provided only a weak foundation for global infectious disease surveillance.

The third conclusion leading WHO in the direction of including non-governmental sources of information in global surveillance flowed from developments in information technologies. The revolution in information technologies, represented by the Internet and electronic mail, contained possibilities for improved public health surveillance apparent to WHO from the earliest days of the IHR revision process. These possibilities existed with governments, as national ministries of health could exploit these technologies for purposes of improving national surveillance data, which could be shared with WHO. But these technologies also offered WHO unprecedented opportunities to mine non-governmental sources of information in order to enhance global surveillance.

In the mid-1990s, NGOs began to harness the potential of new information technologies for disease surveillance purposes, acting as pioneers in this new area of global public health. In 1994, the Program for Monitoring Emerging Diseases (ProMED) launched ProMED-mail, an 'Internet-based reporting system dedicated to rapid and global dissemination of information about outbreaks of infectious diseases that affect human health' (ProMED, 2003). ProMED-mail sought to use 'electronic communications to provide up-to-date and reliable news on disease outbreaks around the world, seven days a week. By providing early warning of outbreaks of emerging and re-emerging diseases, public health precautions at all levels can be taken in a timely manner to prevent epidemic transmission and to save lives' (ProMED, 2003).

ProMED-mail's first e-mail in August 1994 reached 40 subscribers in seven countries; in 2003, ProMED-mail was reaching 30 000 subscribers in over 150 countries (ProMED 2003). Three years after ProMED-mail began, its director emphasized the potential of new information technologies for disease surveillance when he claimed that '[t]he experience of operating ProMED-mail over nearly three years has shown that the public, interactive, unofficial reporting of outbreaks can be faster than through official channels, yet be reliable and responsive to the needs of healthcare providers in epidemic locales' (Woodall, 1997).

The availability and potential of new information technologies provided WHO with new opportunities to improve global infectious disease surveillance by accessing non-governmental sources of information. Prior to the IHR revision process, WHO had access to non-governmental sources of epidemiological information; but, by law, it was very limited in how it could use such information. Legally, the IHR operated only on the basis of government-provided information. Under the IHR, WHO could not disseminate epidemiological information about an outbreak of disease subject to the Regulations that WHO had obtained from a non-governmental source, no matter how reliable. The IHR (1969, Article 11.2) do provide that '[a]ny additional epidemiological data and other information available to the Organization through its surveillance programme shall be made available, when appropriate, to all health administrations.' The scope of the information covered by this provision is, however, tied directly to information provided by governments (Leive, 1976, p. 82).

This legal situation reflected Westphalian limitations on WHO's ability to act independently of formal legal rules and to interfere with sovereignty in connection with infectious diseases. WHO's efforts to establish effective international surveillance suffered from these Westphalian constraints on using epidemiological information. WHO (2002d, p. 3) identified its dependence on notifications from its member states as one of the major constraints of the existing IHR.

Only once during the IHR's history did WHO report an outbreak of a disease subject to the Regulations to the international community based on information not received from the government of the country concerned (Tomasevski, 1995, p. 865). In 1970, Guinea suffered a severe outbreak of cholera. The Guinean government refused to notify WHO of the outbreak, even though it was required to do so under the IHR. Appeals from the WHO Director-General also had no effect in changing the Guinean government's position. Eventually the Director-General publicly disseminated information about the cholera outbreak in Guinea despite having received no information from its government on the outbreak (Leive, 1976, pp. 82–3).

The IHR could not support the Director-General's action, which the Director-General acknowledged in making the Guinea cholera outbreak publicly known (WHO, 1970, p. 1). The Director-General cited Article 2 of the WHO Constitution as the legal justification for his action (WHO, 1970, p. 1). Article 2 of the WHO Constitution lists the functions of the Organization (WHO, 1948). The Director-General argued that WHO could not fulfill its responsibilities under Article 2 without disseminating information about Guinea's cholera outbreak (WHO, 1970, p. 1).

According to Leive (1976, pp. 84–5), four factors explain the Director-General's highly unusual decision. First, WHO was concerned about this severe outbreak in a country not previously exposed to cholera that had poor medical services. Second, WHO had reliable epidemiological information from various sources that cholera had become epidemic in Guinea. Third, WHO had repeatedly tried to get the Guinean government to notify the outbreak under the IHR. Fourth, the Director-General at the time of this incident, M. Candau, was 'extraordinarily widely respected; it is doubtful whether another official without his standing could have taken the same action' (Leive, 1976, p. 84).

WHO's Committee on Communicable Diseases and Executive Board both ratified the Director-General's action concerning the cholera outbreak in Guinea (Leive, 1976, p. 85). The Committee on Communicable Diseases even went as far as to say that 'the Director-General should take similar action in future, should circumstances warrant it, in the interests of all States' (Leive, 1976, p. 85). Leive (1976, p. 85) commented that '[t]he action constitutes an extraordinary invocation by the Director-General of inherent authority to act in a genuine emergency when the interests of WHO in preventing the spread of disease are thwarted.'

This episode is interesting for many reasons, but one clear message it sends is the very tight constraints the Westphalian public health governance model placed on WHO's surveillance capabilities under the IHR. Director-General Candau's circumvention of the IHR was never again repeated, despite WHO member states continuing not to comply with their obligations to report under the IHR. A fifth reason could be added to the reasons for Director-General Candau's action – it was taken against a poor, developing country. The great-power bias of the Westphalian approach would have meant that a similar action would never have been contemplated, let alone implemented, against a stronger, more important country.

The Guinean case helps illustrate, however, the radical nature of WHO's proposal to include within IHR surveillance information gathered from non-governmental sources. Rather than constituting the risky invocation of unstated 'inherent authority' in an emergency context against weak countries, WHO wanted to be able to disseminate, on a routine basis, reliable, verified epidemiological information collected from non-governmental sources with respect to all WHO member states. Another proposal in the IHR revision process – to move from disease-specific reporting to notifications of public health emergencies of international concern (WHO, 2002d, p. 4) – would make access to non-governmental information applicable to a broad range of disease threats.

The proposal to allow WHO to use information from non-governmental sources connects with the global health governance and GPGH concepts explored earlier. Giving WHO access to non-governmental information would make non-state actors formal participants in the most important aspect of governance for infectious diseases, surveillance. By providing epidemiological information directly or indirectly to WHO, non-state actors could trigger a process in which governments and intergovernmental organizations would have to respond. In keeping with the concept of global health governance, the inclusion of non-governmental sources of information would produce *global* as opposed to just *international* surveillance. With the IHR supporting global surveillance, the public health initiative would no longer remain the exclusive province of the sovereign state, contrary to the basic tenets of Westphalian public health as reflected in the IHR.

The proposal to use non-governmental sources of information also connected with the growing policy interest in GPGH. Information can be a classic public good because, as Woodward and Smith (2003, p. 14) observe, '[i]nformation *per se*, such as on health risks and treatment régimes, is *in principle* both non-excludable and non-rival in consumption, at all levels from local to global.' To be a public good, however, information has to be useful to those consuming it. As the IHR's history reveals, the epidemiological information the IHR generated was suspect in quality for two reasons. First, WHO members routinely failed to report epidemiological information the IHR legally required them to report. Second, the short list of diseases subject to the IHR's requirements constrained the range of surveillance information.

The quality of surveillance information as a public good would improve with WHO able to use sources of information beyond governments. WHO's proposal to replace the IHR's limited disease coverage with duties to report the broader category of 'public health emergencies of international concern' would combine with a larger supply of information to improve global surveillance data as a public good. Improved surveillance would be a *global* public good because (1) its production would involve non-state actors as providers and as consumers of information; and (2) its non-excludable, non-rival consumption would extend across national boundaries and traditional regional groupings.

The previous paragraphs do not describe all the ideas WHO proposed in the IHR revision process but focus on the proposal that most represents a post-Westphalian strategy for public health governance. Furthermore, the proposal on use of non-governmental information proved the most compelling IHR revision idea. The potential of transforming international surveillance into global surveillance as envisioned in the IHR revision process was so substantial that WHO began to harvest it early in the process.

WHO began operating its Global Outbreak Alert and Response Network (Global Network) in 1998. The Global Network was expressly designed to collect and analyze information from both governmental and non-governmental sources. WHO (2002d, p. 58) describes the Global Network 'as a mechanism for keeping the volatile microbial world under close surveillance and ensuring that outbreaks are quickly detected and contained. This overarching network interlinks, in real time, 110 existing networks which together possess much of the data, expertise, and skills needed to keep the international community alert to outbreaks and ready to respond.' According to WHO (2003b, p. 4), '[o]ne of the most powerful new tools for gathering epidemiological intelligence is a customized search engine that continuously scans world Internet communications for rumors and reports of suspicious disease events.' This search engine – the Global Public Health Intelligence Network (GPHIN) – was developed by Health Canada, and WHO began to use GPHIN as early as 1997 (WHO, 2003b, p. 4). GPHIN continuously and systematically searches 'web sites, news wires, local online newspapers, public health email services, and electronic discussion groups for rumours of outbreaks' (WHO, 2002a, p. 58). WHO (2003b, pp. 4–5) reports that 'GPHIN currently picks up – in real time – the first hints of about 40% of the roughly 200 to 250 outbreaks subsequently investigated and verified by WHO each year.' GPHIN became an integral component of the Global Network when WHO began operating it in 1998. WHO formally launched the Global Network in 2000 (WHO, 2002a, p. 58).

According to WHO (2003b, p. 4), from January 1998 through March 2002, WHO used the Global Network to identify and investigate 538 outbreaks of international concern in 132 countries. Outbreaks investigated using the Global Network involved diseases not subject to the IHR, including meningitis, haemorrhagic fevers, viral encephalitis, and anthrax (WHO, 2002a, p. 60). The volume of surveillance data gathered, the geographical scope of the surveillance effort, the 'real time' speed of the data collection, and the disease coverage of the network surpass anything ever accomplished under the IHR.

The operation of the Global Network, and its surveillance scope, are astonishing from the perspective of Westphalian public health because the Global Network was operating without formal legal authority or express policy approval from WHO member states. Despite claims that the Global Network operated within the framework of the IHR (Heymann, 2002), the Regulations did not, and could not, support a system of global surveillance that used non-governmental sources of information and covered diseases not subject to the Regulations. The operation of the Global Network ignored the Westphalian tenet of restricting sovereignty only through consent-based rules of international law.

Formal policy recognition and approval of WHO's ability to use non-governmental sources of surveillance information came from the World Health Assembly in 2001, before the IHR revision process was even close to being completed (World Health Assembly, 2001). WHO member states gave their stamp of approval to the post-Westphalian strategy of global surveillance through the Global Network. WHO, backed by its highest policy-making body, moved into global health governance and GPGH production without a specific international legal framework in place – yet another break from the Westphalian model of infectious disease governance.

Post-Westphalian worries

This chapter has demonstrated that, prior to SARS, public health policy had begun to craft and implement post-Westphalian governance strategies on infectious diseases and other public health problems, such as tobacco control. The most well-known infectious-disease strategies – the Global Fund and other public–private partnerships on infectious diseases – owed much to the global disaster HIV/AIDS had become by the end of the twentieth century. The HIV/AIDS pandemic, combined with the recognition of the growing threats of tuberculosis and malaria in the developing world, placed the already troubled Westphalian approach to infectious diseases under intense scrutiny; and it was found wanting. With HIV/AIDS, the post-Westphalian strategies represented increasingly desperate attempts to mitigate a public health nightmare of historic proportions.

The Global Fund was, however, in serious trouble in its first year of operations. In October 2002, *The Economist* reported that '[o]n current projections ... the fund will run out of cash in the second quarter of 2003. And even if it survives that, the projected shortfall in 2004 is $4.6 billion' (*The Economist*, 2002). The Global AIDS Alliance also observed in October 2002 that the Global Fund 'faces de-facto bankruptcy' (Kapp, 2002). In January 2003, the Global Fund announced that it did not have sufficient funds to complete a third round of funding and needed more than $6 billion over the next two years' (Global Fund, 2003e).

With the Global Fund nearly bankrupt after operating for less than two years, concerns were mounting about the sustainability of the new governance approaches to infectious diseases. If the emerging strategies of post-Westphalian public health could not handle the strain existing diseases created, what would happen when the next infectious disease crisis broke upon the world?

Part II

The SARS Outbreak and Post-Westphalian Public Health

5
Brief History of the Global SARS Outbreak of 2002–03

An epidemic unfolds before the global society

Severe Acute Respiratory Syndrome (SARS) was the first severe infectious disease to emerge in the twenty-first century. SARS was also a global epidemic that unfolded with an unprecedented amount of global attention. Even with the war in Iraq taking place during the early phases of the global response, SARS gained significant press and media coverage for weeks. The global community witnessed a world-wide health threat unfold and could watch and follow closely how national and international public health authorities grappled with the outbreak. The surgical mask, worn by citizens of SARS-affected areas, became a global symbol of the threat and the fear that SARS triggered.

This chapter does not attempt a comprehensive history of the SARS outbreak, because such an undertaking would itself produce a book. Rather, this chapter provides a brief narrative history of the SARS outbreak to highlight the key moments, episodes, and developments. My objective is to give the reader a general sense of what happened during the outbreak. This sense will help the reader follow the arguments in Chapters 6–8 more effectively.

Sometime before November 2002: Animal to human, Guangdong Province?

The question on many minds, not least the epidemiologists and public health experts struggling to contain SARS, was: From where did SARS come? Over the course of the outbreak, epidemiological guesses about SARS' origin were made. Although, at the time of this writing, none of the guesses had been definitively proved, the leading hypothesis is that the SARS virus was transmitted from an animal species to humans somewhere in Guangdong Province, China.

Species-jumping pathogens are nothing new in the world of public health. Many of the great disease scourges of human history began when viruses or bacteria were transmitted from animal hosts to human populations. Tuberculosis is, for example, believed to have jumped from animals to humans during the process of human domestication of livestock. Many experts also think that HIV/AIDS originated in simian or primate species before jumping into humans sometime in the twentieth century.

The eventual identification of Guangdong Province as the origin of the species-jumping SARS virus also came as no great surprise for epidemiologists. The southern region of China has long been considered a particularly potent microbial incubator. Guangdong Province is, for example, 'famous for its "wet markets," where a bewildering variety of live fauna are offered for sale (sometimes illegally) for the medicinal properties or culinary potential. The opportunity for contact, not only with farmed animals but also with a variety of otherwise rare or uncommon wild animals, is enormous' (Breiman *et al.*, 2003, p. 1038). This region of China is also important to global surveillance efforts on influenza because of the role experts believe the region's animal–human milieu plays in nurturing strains of the influenza virus.

The southeast Asian region had also been the location of two previous scary but ultimately limited viral outbreaks – the H5N1 avian influenza outbreak in Hong Kong in 1997 and the Nipah virus outbreak in 1998–99 in Malaysia. The H5N1 virus spread from birds to humans, and the Nipah virus spread from pigs to people. Because neither the H5N1 virus nor the Nipah virus developed efficient human-to-human transmission, the outbreaks remained limited in scope and impact. The H5N1 and Nipah viruses constituted, however, warnings that species-jumping viruses were jumping and potentially dangerous. Public health experts have kept an eye on southern China and southeast Asia as a possible, if not the probable, source of the long-anticipated, killer pandemic influenza virus.

In late May 2003, WHO (2003j-2) reported that researchers in Hong Kong and Shenzhen, China announced they had detected several viruses closely related genetically to the SARS virus in two wild animal species, the masked palm civet and the raccoon-dog. The researchers also found antibodies to the SARS virus in another wild animal species, the Chinese ferret badger (WHO, 2003j-2). According to WHO (2003j-2), '[t]hese and other wild animals are traditionally considered delicacies and are sold for human consumption in markets throughout southern China.'

These studies prompted researchers to posit in June 2003 'that the earliest cases of SARS, in Guangdong Province, China, may have had contact, during slaughter or due to proximity to so-called "wet" markets, with certain wild animals species consumed as delicacies in southern China' (WHO, 2003u-2). At the time of this writing, scientists still had not proved or disproved these hypotheses about the origin of SARS. As WHO (2003u-2) argued in June 2003, '[a]dditional studies are urgently needed before any firm conclusions can be reached. Answers to these questions will also greatly assist predictions of the future evolution of SARS.'

November 2002 to February 2003: Outbreak in Guangdong Province

Public health officials are fairly confident, however, that, from a yet to be identified source, the SARS virus emerged in human populations in Guangdong Province sometime prior to or during November 2002. During this month a mysterious outbreak of an atypical respiratory disease occurred. The first SARS case 'is thought to have occurred in Foshan, a city southwest of Guangzhou in Guangdong Province, in mid-November 2002' (Huang, 2003, p. 65). Provincial health authorities and the Ministry of Health in Beijing were aware of, and had investigated, the outbreak in Guangdong Province by the end of January 2003 (Huang, 2003, pp. 65–6). The health authority for Guangdong Province issued a report on cases of atypical pneumonia in the Province on 23 January, but this report was not circulated widely and was not shared with WHO (SARS Expert Committee, 2003, p. 195). The reports written after these investigations were 'top secret' under Chinese law, making any public reporting or discussion of the outbreak a violation of state secrecy laws (Huang, 2003, p. 66). Despite efforts by local and central government officials to suppress news and information about the outbreak, word of the disease problem gradually emerged in an ever-widening arc, propelled by the Internet (Pottinger and Buckman, 2003). Some of the information getting out indicated that, by January 2003, the outbreak in Guangdong Province was causing panic in the population (Pomfret and Goodman, 2003).

WHO's Global Outbreak Alert and Response Network (Global Network) had picked up information about an influenza outbreak in mainland China on 27 November 2002, but the report was never translated into

English at WHO (National Advisory Committee, 2003, p. 24). Further, this early information was full of 'noise' because it did not, at that time, clearly point to an outbreak of an unusual respiratory disease. Early WHO efforts to peg the outbreak focused on influenza or a possible re-emergence of the H5N1 virus (Chase *et al.*, 2003; Stein, 2003f).

The amount of information WHO's Global Network collected about disease problems in southern China increased through early February (Stein, 2003f). According to the *Washington Post*, awareness of the outbreak in Guangdong Province rose to new levels in the days following a mobile phone text message, sent on 8 February, that read: 'There is a fatal flu in Guangzhou' (Pomfret, 2003r). Mobile phone users re-sent this message 40 million times on 8 February, 41 million times on 9 February, and 45 million times on 10 February (Pomfret, 2003r). The same news spread rapidly through e-mail and Internet chat rooms in China and beyond (Pomfret, 2003r). Despite government restrictions on publishing information, journalists in Guangzhou printed stories about the outbreak from 9–11 February (Garrett, 2003). On 10 February, local media published, for example, a circular that 'acknowledged the presence of the disease and listed some preventive measures, including improving ventilation, using vinegar fumes to disinfect the air, and washing hands frequently' (Huang, 2003, p. 67).

On 10 February, ProMED-mail, a leading non-governmental global electronic reporting system for outbreaks of emerging infectious diseases, posted one such e-mail message asking about an epidemic in Guangzhou being linked, in Internet chat rooms, to hospital closings and fatalities (ProMED-mail, 2003). Also on 10 February, the WHO office in Beijing received an alarming e-mail message from the son of a former WHO employee in China, which the office passed along to Dr David Heymann, WHO's Executive Director of Communicable Diseases: 'Am wondering if you have information on the strange contagious disease ... which has already left more than 100 people dead. The outbreak is not allowed to be made known to the public ... but people are already aware ... and there is a "panic" attitude' (Piller, 2003).

WHO made its first official approach to the Chinese government for information on 10 February. On 11 February, the Chinese government made its first report to WHO, notifying the Organization 'of an outbreak of acute respiratory syndrome with 300 cases and five deaths in Guangdong Province' (WHO, 2003c). On the same day, 'Guangdong health officials finally broke the silence by holding press conferences about the disease' (Huang, 2003, p. 67), at which such officials 'informed the public that the situation was under control' (SARS Expert Committee,

2003, p. 196). On 12 February, WHO (2003d) stated that the Chinese Ministry of Health had reported 305 cases and five deaths of acute respiratory syndrome from 16 November 2002 until 9 February 2003. The Chinese Ministry of Health also reported that cases were recorded in six municipalities in Guangdong Province – Foshan, Guanzhou, Heyuan, Jiangmen, Shenzhen, and Zhongshan – but that no new cases had been reported in the past week in three municipalities (Foshan, Heyuan, and Zhongshan) and the number of cases was decreasing in the other three (Guangzhou, Jiangmen, and Shenzhen) (WHO, 2003d). China's communications to WHO clearly indicated that the outbreak was under control and declining. Perhaps this position explains why China declined WHO's offers of assistance to address the outbreak (Pottinger *et al.*, 2003).

By 14 February, China had reported that it had ruled out influenza, anthrax, pulmonary plague, leptospirosis, and haemorrhagic fevers as the source of the respiratory outbreak in Guangdong Province (WHO, 2003d; WHO, 2003e). Into this environment came reports of a possible outbreak of avian influenza in Hong Kong. On 19 February, WHO (2003f) reported that the H5N1 virus had been isolated from a nine-year-old boy from Hong Kong who had traveled to Fujian Province, China in January with his mother and his sisters. The boy's father was admitted to hospital in Hong Kong on 11 February and the boy was admitted on 12 February (SARS Expert Committee, 2003, p. 197). The boy recovered from this illness, as did his mother, but one sister and the father died of illness on 4 February and 17 February, respectively (WHO, 2003f; SARS Expert Committee, 2003, p. 197). On 19 February, WHO noted that it did not know whether the boy's family members who fell ill had been infected by the H5N1 virus. WHO put its Global Influenza Surveillance Network on alert (WHO, 2003f). On 20 February, WHO (2003g) disclosed that the father who died on 17 February had been infected by the H5N1 virus.

These cases of avian influenza raised the question of whether the outbreak of atypical respiratory disease in Guangdong Province was caused by the H5N1 virus. The Chinese Ministry of Health informed WHO on 20 February, however, that the probable causative agent of the Guangdong outbreak was *Chlamydia pneumoniae* (WHO, 2003h). Government officials imposed another blackout on reporting news of the outbreak on 23 February (Huang, 2003, p. 67). By 27 February, WHO (2003i) reported that the Chinese Ministry of Health had declared the outbreak in Guangdong Province over and that no evidence existed to link the Guangdong situation with the H5N1 cases in Hong Kong. As late as 7 March, however, WHO still had not completely excluded the H5N1 virus as the cause of the Guangdong outbreak (SARS Expert Committee, 2003, p. 201).

February 2003: Guangdong, Hong Kong, Hanoi

In mid-February 2003, Dr Liu Jianlun, a professor of nephrology at Zhongshan University in Guangzhou, Guangdong Province, had been treating patients suffering from atypical pneumonia at a hospital in Guangdong Province (Pottinger, 2003a). On 21 February, despite feeling feverish, Dr Liu arrived in Hong Kong to attend his nephew's wedding (Pottinger, 2003a; SARS Expert Committee, 2003, p. 198; National Advisory Committee, 2003, p. 24). Dr Liu stayed on the ninth floor, Room 911, of the Metropole Hotel in Hong Kong for one night (WHO, 2003e-1; Pottinger, 2003a; SARS Expert Committee, 2003, p. 198). Dr Liu was admitted to a Hong Kong hospital on 22 February with severe pneumonia, and he died on 4 March (SARS Expert Committee, 2003, p. 18). Experts believe that Dr Liu was infected with SARS-CoV and that, during his brief stay on the ninth floor of the Metropole Hotel, he communicated the virus to at least 16 other guests and visitors to the same floor of the hotel, including a resident of Hong Kong, an American national with business interests in Vietnam, Singaporean nationals, and two Canadian nationals (WHO, 2003e-1; WHO 2003g-3; Pottinger, 2003a). The seeds of a global epidemic were planted on the ninth floor of the Metropole Hotel.

The American businessman who stayed on the ninth floor of the Metropole Hotel at the same time as Dr Liu, Johnny Chen, traveled to Hanoi, Vietnam after finishing his visit to Hong Kong. Mr Chen fell ill in Hanoi in late February 2003 (Cohen, Fritsch, and Pottinger, 2003). He was taken to the Hanoi French Hospital, where his condition worsened. Dr Olivier Cattin, a physician at the Hanoi French Hospital, wondered whether Mr Chen's severe respiratory illness could be avian influenza connected to the outbreaks of the H5N1 virus he had heard about in Hong Kong earlier in the month (Cohen, Naik, and Pottinger, 2003). Mr Chen had come to Hanoi from Hong Kong.

Dr Cattin consulted with Dr Carlo Urbani, a WHO epidemiologist in Hanoi. Dr Urbani is credited with being the first to identify that the illness affecting Mr Chen was a new disease syndrome (WHO, 2003w). Dr Urbani made this diagnosis on 28 February (Cohen, Naik, and Pottinger, 2003). Dr Urbani's worries about Mr Chen's ailment escalated as hospital staff at the Hanoi French Hospital began falling ill with symptoms that mirrored the mysterious respiratory condition affecting Mr Chen (WHO, 2003l).

March 2003: A world-wide health threat

Dr Urbani's 28 February diagnosis of an unknown severe respiratory syndrome proved the trigger for a cascade of events that led WHO to take drastic action. As more staff at the Hanoi French Hospital fell ill, Dr Urbani communicated his concerns about Mr Chen's illness and the apparent spread of the syndrome among hospital staff to the Vietnamese government and his WHO colleagues. Difficult and heated talks with Vietnamese government officials on 9 March led to Vietnam agreeing to take the aggressive measures prescribed by Urbani and his WHO colleagues for the situation in Hanoi (Cohen, Naik, and Pottinger, 2003; Nakashima, 2003b). By 10 March, approximately 20 staff at the Hanoi French Hospital had become ill with the same syndrome Dr Urbani diagnosed in Mr Chen (WHO, 2003j). Dr Urbani told Dr Klaus Stöhr, a WHO influenza specialist, that 'we're losing control of the hospital' (Cohen, Naik, and Pottinger, 2003). Dr Urbani's actions helped prime WHO for the events about to break upon the Organization and the world.

Alarm bells at WHO began ringing loudly on 12 March when Hong Kong reported an outbreak of a severe respiratory illness at one of its public hospitals (WHO, 2003j; SARS Expert Committee, 2003, p. 203). Hong Kong's hospital authority had noticed that an unusually high number of medical staff at the Prince of Wales Hospital were not reporting to work because of suffering from a flu-like illness (Cohen, Naik, and Pottinger, 2003). By 12 March, the situation was severe enough for Hong Kong's health director to call WHO (Cohen, Naik, and Pottinger, 2003). WHO faced the possibility that the Guangdong, Hanoi, and Hong Kong outbreaks were connected. If these outbreaks were related, WHO would be facing a severe new respiratory disease that had already demonstrated cross-border mobility.

On 12 March, WHO issued a global alert about cases of atypical pneumonia (WHO, 2003j). The decision proved difficult for many reasons, including the unprecedented nature of the decision. WHO's Mike Ryan remembered: 'We wondered: "Are we mad? Are we going to panic the world?"' (Cohen, Naik, and Pottinger, 2003). In the alert, WHO disclosed the hospital outbreaks in Hanoi and Hong Kong and provided a description of the symptoms the illness appeared to present in patients. WHO recommended that medical staff isolate patients with atypical pneumonia who may be connected to the Hanoi or Hong Kong outbreaks through barrier nursing techniques. WHO also recommended that any suspect cases be reported to national authorities. The global alert sought to raise the level of epidemiological awareness around the world given the unknown nature and scope of the new severe respiratory syndrome.

The global alert on 12 March was carefully worded to avoid linking the Guangdong, Hanoi, and Hong Kong outbreaks. The alert stated, for example, that 'no link has been found between these [Hong Kong] cases and the outbreak in Hanoi' (WHO, 2003j). The careful wording could not hide WHO's concern that these three outbreaks were related. WHO wanted to express this concern without making statements the epidemiological data could not yet support. The alert began: 'Since mid-February, WHO has been actively working to confirm reports of outbreaks of a severe form of pneumonia in Vietnam, Hong Kong Special Administrative Region (SAR), China, and Guangdong Province in China' (WHO, 2003j).

In the days immediately following the global alert of 12 March, WHO began receiving reports of cases of severe atypical respiratory illnesses from multiple countries. By 15 March, WHO received information on more than 150 new suspected cases of atypical pneumonia for which a cause had not been identified from Canada, China, Hong Kong, Indonesia, the Philippines, Singapore, and Vietnam (WHO, 2003k). Although the reports of such cases to WHO indicated that the 12 March global alert had increased awareness around the world about possible cases of unusual respiratory illnesses, the reports also provided evidence that an international outbreak was underway.

In the early morning hours of 15 March, Singapore urgently notified WHO of a Singaporean physician with symptoms of atypical pneumonia on board a flight from New York to Singapore, with a stopover in Frankfurt, Germany (WHO, 2003b, p. 3). WHO worked with German officials to remove the physician and accompanying family members, who were immediately isolated and given hospital care (WHO, 2003b, p. 3).

Later on 15 March, in light of these developments, and after difficult discussions among its infectious disease experts, WHO issued another global alert, this time in the form of an emergency travel advisory (WHO, 2003k). This decision was riskier politically than the 12 March global alert because it linked the spread of the mysterious syndrome with air travel, making the 15 March alert 'a decision that would have huge implications for world business and tourism' (Cohen, Naik, and

Pottinger, 2003). Given the lack of much information about the syndrome and its characteristics, some of WHO's infectious disease experts worried about the impact on WHO if the emergency travel advisory proved a mistake or an over-reaction (Cohen, Naik, and Pottinger, 2003). Eventually, the arguments in favor of issuing the emergency travel advisory carried the day.

By this point, WHO was certain that the new illness was not influenza (Chase *et al.*, 2003). In this alert, WHO gave the new illness a name – Severe Acute Respiratory Syndrome, or SARS. WHO Director-General Gro Harlem Brundtland stated in the alert that '[t]his syndrome, SARS[,] is now a worldwide health threat. The world needs to work together to find its cause, cure the sick, and stop its spread' (WHO, 2003k).

The 15 March global alert made no recommendations that people restrict their travel to any destination reporting SARS cases. WHO provided, however, information on the symptoms and signs of SARS to assist travelers, airlines, physicians, and governments. The global alert described the removal and subsequent isolation of the Singaporean physician and family members on the flight from New York to Frankfurt. Although air travel was clearly playing a role in spreading SARS, WHO's emergency guidance to travelers and airlines did not expressly address the possibility that SARS may be transmitted during flights. The global alert repeated WHO's recommendations that patients with suspected cases of SARS be isolated with barrier infection-control techniques and treated clinically as indicated and that all suspect cases be reported to national health authorities.

WHO now had the task of leading and coordinating the investigation and containment of an international epidemic of a new respiratory syndrome. A central function of WHO's responsibility for this task was acting as a clearing-house for surveillance data on SARS and for information on the best public health and clinical approaches to containing the syndrome and treating those afflicted. On 16 March, WHO (2003l) issued the first of many updates on the multi-country outbreak of SARS, as the Organization quickly took the lead on SARS surveillance and response efforts.

The 16 March update reported what WHO had learned about the epidemiology of SARS. The causative agent was not known, and the syndrome appeared to be transmissible from person-to-person through aerosol and/or droplet means as well as through bodily fluids. WHO reported that the majority of SARS cases to date had occurred in individuals who had very close contact with persons already infected with SARS, such as health care personnel and family members. Over 90 per cent of SARS cases had occurred in health care workers. The 16 March update provided those handling SARS cases with more technical guidance for this task. It contained Internet jump links to two documents: (1) Hospital Infection Control Guidance for Severe Acute Respiratory Syndrome (SARS); and (2) Management of Severe Acute Respiratory Syndrome (SARS). WHO would continue to revise this technical guidance as the epidemiology of SARS became better understood.

The 16 March update also contained information about the status of the SARS outbreak in the countries believed affected. Table 5.1 summarizes this initial data. From this date forward, WHO posted on its website a daily summary of reported cases of SARS.

Conspicuously missing from the list of countries reporting suspected cases of SARS was China. As noted earlier, suspicions about the possible link between the Guangdong outbreak of November 2002–February 2003 and the various outbreaks now categorized as SARS had been strong. In connection to China, the 16 March update tersely stated: 'An epidemic of atypical pneumonia had previously been reported by the Chinese government starting in November 2002 in Guangdong Province. This epidemic is reported to be under control' (WHO, 2003l).

On 17 March, WHO (2003m) reported that China had issued a report summarizing 'an outbreak of what may be the same or a related disease that began in Guangdong Province in November and peaked in mid-February.' This summary report did not, apparently, provide any updated information because it only included data on the diagnosis and management of the 300 cases reported by China in February. WHO also reported on 17 March that China had requested help from an

Table 5.1 SARS outbreak data as of 15 March 2003

Country	*Suspected cases*	*Deaths*
Vietnam (Hanoi)	43	2
Hong Kong	100	1
Singapore	16	0
Thailand	1	0
Canada	7	2
Philippines	1*	0
Indonesia	1*	0
Germany	1*	0

Note: *Unconfirmed case
Source: WHO 2003l

international team and that WHO was assembling the requested assistance (WHO, 2003m; Carrns *et al.*, 2003).

With health authorities around the world alerted to the SARS threat, and with reporting of cases from around the world happening, for the most part, openly and rapidly, WHO moved to ramp up the scientific and epidemiological investigation of SARS. Through its Global Network, WHO began on 17 March to coordinate a global scientific effort involving eleven laboratories in 10 countries to identify the pathogen causing SARS (WHO, 2003m; Stein, 2003a). This unprecedented scientific collaboration sought to locate the causative agent for SARS and filter that basic scientific research into the development of diagnostic technologies for SARS.

This global scientific effort produced preliminary findings, which WHO released on 18 March, that suggested that the causative agent behind SARS was a virus from the paramyxoviridae family (WHO, 2003n; Stein, 2003b). Viruses in this family are often associated with respiratory infections and include the mumps and measles viruses. The paramyxoviridae family also includes the Nipah virus, which emerged in Malaysia in 1998 causing 265 deaths (WHO, 2003o). The Nipah virus did not, however, establish human-to-human transmission (WHO, 2003o). The causative agent of SARS had established such transmission between persons with the syndrome and those in very close contact with them, such as health care personnel and family members. Whatever was causing SARS was, thus, more dangerous to global public health than the Nipah virus but not yet exhibiting the more potent human-to-human transmissibility of viruses such as influenza or smallpox. WHO stressed, however, that preliminary scientific findings suggesting a paramyxovirus did not represent definitive success in locating the SARS pathogen (WHO, 2003o).

WHO continued building global networks to help with the response to SARS. To its Global Network for surveillance and response and its global SARS laboratory network, WHO instituted an unprecedented global network of clinicians to share information and experiences on the diagnosis and treatment of SARS (WHO, 2003p). WHO (2003p) reported on 20 March that the 'network brings together, via two daily teleconferences, clinicians in the most heavily affected Asian countries and in Europe and North America.' These global 'electronic grand rounds' (Stein, 2003c) were designed to disseminate globally and rapidly best practices on SARS diagnosis and treatment as an integral element of the overall effort to contain the spread of SARS and the suffering it inflicted on the infected (WHO, 2003p). The WHO official in charge of the effort, Mark Salter, told the *Washington Post* that '[t]he WHO has never brought together this many clinicians with such rapidity. It's ground-breaking' (Stein, 2003c).

Efforts to trace the origins of the multi-country outbreak were also bearing some fruit. On 20 March, WHO (2003p) reported the release of Hong Kong's investigation of the 'index' case of the SARS outbreak in Hong Kong. Hong Kong's index case was an acquaintance of Dr Liu Jianlun, the professor-physician from Guangdong Province, who met with Dr Liu in the Metropole Hotel during Dr Liu's February stay in Hong Kong (WHO, 2003p). Johnny Chen, the American businessman who contracted SARS while at the Metropole and who sparked the outbreak in Hanoi, also was the source for the outbreak in Hong Kong's Princess Margaret Hospital, to which Mr Chen had transferred from Hanoi (WHO, 2003e-1).

In addition, the Hong Kong epidemiologists found the source of SARS infection in other people – three from Singapore and two from Canada – connected to the Metropole Hotel and Dr Liu (WHO, 2003p). Singapore's initial report of SARS cases on 13 March involved the three persons who returned to Singapore after visiting Hong Kong and staying at the Metropole Hotel (WHO, 2003l). Canada's initial cluster of cases was traced back to the two Canadians who stayed at the Metropole Hotel in Hong Kong (WHO, 2003p). All were individuals who either stayed on, or visited, the ninth floor of the Metropole Hotel between 12 February and 2 March (WHO, 2003p).

These investigations began to give the multi-country outbreaks of SARS an epidemiological profile that pointed directly at Guangdong Province in China. The index cases for the SARS outbreaks in Hong Kong, Vietnam, Canada, and Singapore all traced back to a Chinese medical professional from Guangdong Province who traveled to Hong Kong with a fever after treating patients suffering from serious atypical pneumonia. The suspected connection between the Guangdong outbreak and the SARS epidemic now began to solidify.

As WHO (2003q) stated on 21 March, '[t]he outbreak in southern China is linked geographically and by timing to the current outbreak of Severe Acute Respiratory Syndrome (SARS) which first surfaced in Asia in mid-February and caused its first known death on 13 March.' Said WHO's Meirion Evans on 27 March about the link between the Guangdong and SARS outbreaks: 'Everything we've seen so far indicates it's the same disease' (Wonacott, Borsuk, and Cohen, 2003).

The importance of China to the global efforts on SARS increased. A WHO team left for China after 21 March to assist Chinese authorities with their investigation of the Guangdong outbreak (WHO, 2003q).

That same day, the *Washington Post* reported statements from Chinese doctors challenging the government's claims that the outbreak of atypical pneumonia had been contained in Guangdong Province (Pomfret and Goodman, 2003). The initial meetings between the WHO team and Chinese health officials on 24 March did not go well (Cohen, Naik, and Pottinger, 2003). On 25 March, the *Washington Post* reported that WHO officials in Beijing were indicating that information they had been given was insufficient and were pressing Chinese officials for more information (Pomfret, 2003a).

WHO's global laboratory network continued to function productively, achieving isolation of the virus causing SARS and making progress on the development of diagnostic technologies (WHO, 2003r). Although scientists had not yet agreed what kind of virus they had isolated, WHO officials working on the epidemic were heartened by the nature and speed of the global scientific collaboration. The pace of the scientific effort revealed not only how far microbiology had come since HIV emerged in the early 1980s but also the spirit of global collaboration exhibited in the effort (Chase *et al.*, 2003). James Hughes, director of the CDC's National Center for Infectious Diseases, noted that the global collaboration of the scientific laboratories was 'historic. The laboratories around the world – which at other times might be competing with each other to be first to sort this out – are sharing all their information on a daily basis as it's developing, and that's why we're able to make as rapid progress as we have made' (Chase *et al.*, 2003).

Further progress was made as the global scientific network rapidly zeroed in on the identity of the culprit virus. On 26 March, WHO (2003t) indicated that researchers were increasingly focusing on the coronavirus family. The next day, WHO (2003u) reported that data produced by the global scientific network pointed to a coronavirus as the causative pathogen for SARS (SARS-CoV). WHO epidemiologist Klaus Stöhr described SARS-CoV as 'unlike any known human or animal member of the virus family' (WHO, 2003u).

As March began to draw to a close, the global response to SARS appeared to be off to a good start. The *Washington Post* opined that '[t]he international response has been better than many expected, reflecting a number of positive changes within the World Health Organization over the past decade' (*Washington Post*, 2003a). WHO had taken rapid and unprecedented actions that had produced encouraging results in terms of surveillance, response, epidemiological findings, and basic scientific research. Former CDC Director Jeffrey Koplan complimented WHO by observing 'here's a group that acted forcefully and quickly'

(Cohen, Naik, and Pottinger, 2003). Further, compared to the highly efficient person-to-person transmissibility of influenza, the SARS outbreak was, according to WHO, 'not rampaging' (Pottinger and Buckman, 2003). All was not well, however, in the global campaign against SARS. At least three problems confronted the effort.

First, SARS outbreaks continued to grow in virtually all the countries in which SARS-CoV had established a foothold and a chain of human-to-human transmission. Thus, the outbreaks in Hong Kong, Singapore, and Canada grew larger as March progressed. Only Vietnam appeared to have contained its SARS problem during March. On 29 March, WHO (2003w) reported that '[t]he number of cases in Vietnam remained at 58 for the sixth day in a row, indicating that the outbreak in Hanoi is well-controlled.'

The continued growth of the epidemics in Hong Kong, Singapore, and Canada meant that public health authorities had not yet been successful at breaking the chain of human-to-human transmission. Although epidemiological data still indicated that very close contact with a person with SARS was required for transmission, some developments suggested that transmission outside health care facilities may become a problem. Fear of SARS transmission on aircraft grew during March, fueled by reports that people had contracted SARS while passengers on aircraft (Pottinger, 2003b; Stein and Brown, 2003). WHO (2003s) addressed these concerns on 25 March, when it reported information from Hong Kong about passengers on a Beijing tour who had developed atypical pneumonia. WHO (2003s) commented that, '[a]s "close" contact is possible during a flight, in passengers sitting close to an infected person, such transmission cannot be ruled out. The evidence to date indicates that in-flight transmission is very unusual.'

A second transmission scare happened in Hong Kong at the end of March when Hong Kong authorities issued unprecedented isolation orders against residents of the Amoy Gardens apartment building (Pomfret and Weiss, 2003). The isolation orders sought to break a chain of SARS transmission in Amoy Gardens, a transmission pattern in the community different from the dominant health care transmission setting. Eventually the Amoy Gardens outbreak affected 329 residents with 42 deaths (SARS Expert Committee, 2003, p. 40). Both this episode and the concerns about SARS transmission on aircraft suggested that more work on SARS' epidemiology was needed, despite the progress that had been rapidly made. Neither of these developments persuaded WHO, however, to change its position that travel to, and travel from, SARS-affected areas was not dangerous.

The second problem confronting the global effort against SARS at the end of March was the syndrome's continued international spread. By the end of March, WHO was receiving reports of SARS cases from 13 countries (WHO, 2003x). Although WHO's global alerts and recommendations helped most countries prevent onward transmission of imported SARS cases, WHO remained concerned about international travel as a means of spreading SARS. Of significant concern for WHO was the prospect of SARS importation into developing countries that did not have very strong public health systems. On 20 March, WHO (2003p) noted that '[u]p to now, all imported cases have occurred in countries well-equipped and well-prepared to institute WHO-recommended precautions, including isolation and barrier nursing practices, for preventing spread to others, whether healthcare workers or family members.' This circumstance positively affected the SARS response to date. But even these well-equipped and well-prepared countries were struggling to contain SARS transmission. WHO was concerned about the potential impact on global SARS efforts if human-to-human transmission of SARS got underway in poor, less well-prepared nations.

Evidence of WHO's growing concerns about SARS spreading through international travel came on 27 March, when WHO issued new recommendations to prevent travel-related spread of SARS (Pomfret, 2003c). WHO (2003u) recommended that authorities in areas experiencing human-to-human transmission of SARS institute the screening of air passengers departing the affected areas in flights to other countries. As of 27 March, these recommendations affected only four countries – Hong Kong, Singapore, Vietnam, and Canada; but WHO's issuance of the recommendations demonstrated WHO's growing concern about international travel spreading SARS from countries that had not yet broken the chain of human-to-human transmission.

The third major problem for the WHO-led global SARS effort was China. Although the epidemiological link between the Guangdong outbreak and the SARS outbreak was strong, China did not provide WHO with updated data on the Guangdong outbreak between its initial report on 10 February and 25 March. On 26 March, China reported to WHO new figures in the November–February outbreak in Guangdong Province – 792 cases and 31 deaths from an atypical pneumonia (WHO, 2003o; Pomfret, 2003b). The WHO team invited to help the Chinese government concluded that the atypical pneumonia cases reported were cases of SARS, but Chinese officials 'seemed wedded to the notion that the outbreak was caused by a rare respiratory strain of Chlamydia bacteria' (Cohen, Naik, and Pottinger, 2003). The new Chinese data only covered a period from 16 November 2002 until 28 February 2003. At this point, it was the end of March; and WHO had no data from China for nearly a month, a month in which SARS had become a world-wide health threat.

With the Guangdong outbreak now definitely identified as SARS, China became the country with the largest number of reported cases. The initial task was to update Chinese data for March and get China to improve its surveillance and reporting for SARS. WHO needed to know whether, as China claimed, the Guangdong outbreak had been controlled and was over, or whether Guangdong Province and perhaps other areas of China were 'hot zones' for SARS.

As March wound down, some signs of improved Chinese cooperation appeared. China notified WHO of SARS cases outside Guangdong Province as of 26 March: ten cases and three deaths in Beijing and four cases with no deaths in Shanxi (WHO, 2003u). China pledged to improve its reporting system (WHO, 2003t), contribute to the global scientific effort to identify the causative agent of SARS (WHO, 2003t), participate in the global network on SARS diagnosis and treatment (WHO, 2003v), provide WHO access to Chinese medical records on SARS cases (WHO, 2003v), enhance surveillance in Beijing, gear up laboratory capability, set up a public hotline, and to continue contact tracing (WHO, 2003x). These steps were victories for WHO, 'which has walked a fine line between trying to pressure China for more information and encouraging cooperation' (Pomfret, 2003d).

Ominously, however, the request of the WHO team in Beijing to travel to Guangdong Province to investigate the outbreak there had not been approved by the end of March. WHO officials told the Chinese that '[i]f SARS is not under control in China, there would be little chance of controlling the global threat of the disease' (Cohen, Naik, and Pottinger, 2003). WHO (2003x) diplomatically noted in the final SARS update of March 2003 that '[d]iscussions concerning a visit by the [WHO] expert team to Guangdong Province are continuing with the Ministry of Health.'

On 29 March, Dr Carlo Urbani, the WHO epidemiologist in Hanoi who first identified SARS and helped alert WHO of this new threat, died from his SARS infection (Stein, 2003f). His death was a particularly painful reminder to those still fighting SARS that, by the end of March, the global effort had reached not the beginning of the end of the struggle, but only the end of the beginning.

April 2003: The crisis deepens

On 1 April 2003, WHO (2003y) reported that it had received notifications of 1804 cases of SARS with 62 deaths from 15 countries. On the last day of April 2003, the numbers had risen to 5663 cases with 372 deaths reported from 26 countries (WHO, 2003t-1). For the global SARS campaign, April was the cruelest month. But, it was also the campaign's finest hour.

The deepening of the SARS crisis in April can be attributed to three factors: (1) problems created by continuing questions about the epidemiology of SARS and its causative agent; (2) the threat posed to international travel by SARS 'hot zones'; and (3) the behavior of the country at the epicenter of the global outbreak, China. Led by WHO, the global effort against SARS had to confront each of these major problems during April; and, in two of these cases, WHO faced decisions unprecedented in its history of fighting infectious diseases.

In terms of the epidemiology of SARS, April 2003 witnessed the definitive scientific demonstration that the new coronavirus identified in March was indeed the causative agent of SARS. On 16 April, WHO (2003k-1) announced that its global network of collaborating laboratories had finished putting the identified coronavirus through the tests known as 'Koch's postulates,' which epidemiologists believe provide the definitive tests for whether a microbial agent causes disease. The final steps – introducing the coronavirus into animal hosts, which subsequently develop the disease – confirmed scientifically what experts had begun to suspect when the global laboratory network first identified the new coronavirus. WHO was excited about these developments and noted that the 'astounding pace' of scientific research on SARS-CoV strengthens the global effort against the syndrome by providing key information and tools scientists could use in creating technologies for SARS prevention and control (WHO, 2003k-1).

Despite the accomplishment of identifying the new coronavirus and confirming it as the causative agent of SARS, the global SARS effort confronted difficult epidemiological challenges that indicated that much of how SARS-CoV caused illness in humans and spread in populations was not clear. Although the lack of such knowledge was hardly surprising given how recently the outbreak began, the questions meant that WHO and others battling the spread of SARS often did not have answers for pressing questions.

A key quest, undertaken by the global network of scientific laboratories, was to develop diagnostic technologies that would allow public health officials and health care workers to identify with more precision people infected with SARS-CoV. More precise diagnostics would allow more discriminating and effective public health and health care responses. As WHO (2003l-1) argued, '[w]ithout a more reliable diagnostic tool, hospital staff confronted with a suspect SARS case have no option other than to isolate patients and manage them according to strict infection control practices as precautionary measures. Such measures are stressful for patients and place a considerable stain on health services.' But, as WHO (2003g-1) noted on 11 April, '[t]he development of a diagnostic test has proved more problematic than hoped.' Each of the three tests developed, to that point, had significant shortcomings.

The ELISA test provided reliable results but only after the onset of clinical symptoms of SARS, meaning that the test could not be used to detect cases at an earlier stage before infected persons had a chance to spread the virus (WHO, 2003g-1). The immunofluorescence assay (IFA) test gave results earlier in a SARS infection but was a slow test requiring the growth of SARS-CoV in cell culture (WHO, 2003g-1). The PCR molecular test proved useful for even earlier stages of a SARS infection but unfortunately produced many false-negatives, making it unreliable as a diagnostic tool (WHO, 2003g-1). In the absence of good diagnostic technologies, diagnosis of SARS remained focused on clinical symptoms, history of the infected (especially recent travel history), and chest X-rays (WHO, 2003g-1). At the end of April 2003, WHO (2003q-1) strongly advised national authorities 'to continue to base decisions concerning what constitutes a suspect and a probable case of SARS on the present clinical and epidemiological case definition, and not to rely on the results of diagnostic tests.'

A second set of epidemiological questions that plagued the global SARS effort in April 2003 revolved around the transmission of SARS-CoV. Although WHO knew that intimate contact with SARS patients was a primary means of transmission of the disease, WHO was concerned that, in some areas, such as Hong Kong and Canada, SARS continued to spread both within health care settings and in the community despite the use of strict patient isolation and infection-control techniques (WHO, 2003g-1). In connection with Hong Kong, the SARS outbreak at the Amoy Gardens apartment complex demonstrated that spread of SARS-CoV in the community from an environmental source could efficiently occur (WHO, 2003n-1). Further, data indicated that infections connected to the Amoy Gardens outbreak were more serious than non-Amoy infections, raising questions of whether the Amoy Gardens cases 'represent infection with high virus loads, as might occur following exposure to a concentrated environmental source, or whether the virus may have mutated into a more virulent form' (WHO, 2003n-1).

In connection with Canada, WHO (2003n-1) expressed concern about suspect and probable SARS cases related to a charismatic religious group, the health care workers who treated them, and close family and social contacts. WHO (2003n-1) noted that this 'outbreak is particularly disturbing because of its potential to move into the wider community.' Questions surrounding this Canadian outbreak connected to speculation that some of the worst situations involving SARS stem from so-called 'super-spreaders.'

WHO (2003f-1) raised the 'super-spreader' concept on 9 April in discussing the outbreak in Singapore. WHO (2003h-1) traced SARS outbreaks at two Singaporean hospitals to a single 'super-spreader'. WHO (2003f-1) defined a super-spreader as 'a source case who has, for as yet unknown reasons, infected a large number of persons.' WHO (2003g-1) noted that '[i]t remains unknown whether such "super-spreaders" are persons secreting an exceptionally high amount of infectious material or whether some other factor, perhaps in the environment, is working to amplify transmission at some key phase of virus shedding.' Cautioning that SARS transmission patterns remain only partly understood, WHO (2003f-1) commented that 'evidence suggests that such "super-spreaders" may have contributed to the evolution of SARS outbreaks around the world.'

Skepticism emerged, however, about the 'super-spreader' concept (Saywell, 2003). The main reasons for the skepticism involved the lack of scientific evidence for the phenomenon and the existence of alternative, more plausible explanations for high infection rates being associated with individual cases. The most plausible alternative was that the 'super-spreader' phenomenon had less to do with a particular individual shedding virus at especially high rates and more to do with the non-application or misapplication of infection control techniques at critical times. As WHO (2003j-1) commented on 15 April, 'when SARS was just becoming known as a severe new disease, many patients were thought to be suffering from atypical pneumonia having another cause, and were therefore not treated as special cases requiring special precautions of isolation and infection control.... Since infection control measures have been put in place, the number of new cases of SARS arising from a single SARS source case has been significantly reduced.'

The diagnostic and 'super-spreader' problems illustrate that the global campaign against SARS was operating in April 2003 under serious constraints involving a lack of basic information about the epidemiology of SARS and appropriate technologies to guide more precise and effective interventions. The continued growth of the SARS outbreak, both within most SARS-affected countries and through international travel, exacerbated the difficulties WHO and its collaborating partners faced in getting SARS under control.

The second major factor deepening the SARS crisis in April 2003 concerned the spread of SARS through international travel. At the beginning of April, WHO's Hitoshi Oshitani stated that SARS was 'the most significant outbreak that has been spread through air travel in history' (Pomfret, 2003e). Until the beginning of April 2003, WHO had not recommended that travelers postpone travel to SARS-affected areas, maintaining that outbreaks were confined to specific settings, such as health care facilities, and were not threats to public health in the community. As SARS continued to spread within SARS 'hot zones,' such as Hong Kong and Guangdong Province, WHO became more and more concerned about travelers visiting these destinations, contracting SARS, and spreading it to their countries of origin upon their return home. WHO's worries on this issue became so severe that it took actions unprecedented in the history of the Organization.

At the end of March 2003, as mentioned above, WHO (2003u) recommended that airport authorities in SARS-affected areas screen passengers leaving for other countries for potential symptoms of SARS. These recommendations were indications of WHO's growing fears about the spread of SARS through international travel. On 3 April, WHO (2003z) issued recommendations 'that persons traveling to Hong Kong and Guangdong Province of China consider postponing non-essential travel.' According to WHO (2003a-1), '[t]he new travel advisory is intended to limit the spread of SARS by reducing travel to high risk areas.' As WHO (2003b-1) noted, '[t]his is the first time in the history of WHO that such travel advice has been issued for specific geographical areas because of an outbreak of an infectious disease.'

As the outbreak at the Amoy Gardens suggested, WHO had being growing increasingly concerned about the pattern of SARS transmission in Hong Kong; and evidence developed at the beginning of April that heightened WHO's worries. WHO partly based its decision to recommend that non-essential travel to Hong Kong be postponed because, 'since March 19, nine travellers have been identified as SARS cases on returning from a visit to Hong Kong Special Administrative Region of China' (WHO, 2003a-1). WHO (2003b-1) observed that '[t]he data on these cases, and what is known about the incubation period of SARS, indicate that travel to Hong Kong can contribute to the international spread of SARS.'

In terms of the travel recommendations against non-essential travel to Guangdong Province, WHO (2003a-1) emphasized that its decision was influenced by '[n]ew information provided today [2 April 2003] by [Chinese] provincial authorities of more than 300 new cases in March alone [, which] indicates the outbreak there continues.' WHO (2003b-1) also focused on the fact that the outbreak in Guangdong Province 'has also shown evidence of spread in the wider community' and spread across international borders. WHO (2003g-1) also justified its advisory on Guangdong Province by asserting that the 'recommendations were made for Guangdong as maximum security against spread of SARS outside of Guangdong in the absence of a complete understanding of transmission patterns of the outbreak there.' As with Hong Kong, WHO perceived that the 'hot zone' in Guangdong Province was sufficiently dangerous to warrant advising non-essential travelers to avoid the province until the outbreak was under control.

Prior to WHO's recommendations against non-essential travel to Hong Kong and Guangdong Province, national governments, such as Canada and the United States, had issued travel advisories encouraging their nationals to postpone non-essential travel to SARS-affected areas (Stein, 2003d; Stein and Brown, 2003). For example, on 29 March, the CDC warned US nationals against unnecessary travel to all of China, Singapore, Hanoi and Hong Kong (Stein, 2003e). Until 2 April, such national-level recommendations did not accord with WHO's advice on travel to these locations.

The issuance of such travel advisories by national governments did not constitute, however, radical acts of sovereign governments. WHO's actions with respect to travel to Hong Kong and Guangdong Province were radical steps for the Organization. As illustrated by complaints from the Chinese government about the travel advisories (Pomfret, 2003f), WHO did not issue the recommendations with the express permission of China. WHO's decisions represented, therefore, independent acts that carried potentially adverse economic consequences for Hong Kong and Guangdong Province. In the travel advisories, WHO wielded considerable authority and power vis-à-vis Hong Kong and Guangdong Province.

An indication of the deepening SARS crisis in April 2003 is the further issuance of travel advisories against two other SARS 'hot zones' toward the end of April. On 23 April, WHO (2003p-1) extended its recommendations against non-essential travel to Beijing and Shanxi Province in China and Toronto, Canada. WHO based these decisions on the following criteria: 'the magnitude of the outbreak, including both the number of prevalent cases and the daily number of new cases, the extent of local chains of transmission, and evidence that travellers are becoming infected while in one area and then subsequently exporting the disease elsewhere' (WHO, 2003p-1). WHO asserted that the 'travel advice is issued in order to protect public health and reduce opportunities for further international spread' (WHO, 2003p-1).

The power of WHO travel advisories, and the controversy they could provoke, both became apparent in the reaction of the Canadian government to the advisory against Toronto: 'the reaction of Canadian officials was swift and angry, with politicians and public health officials from multiple levels of government travelling to Geneva to provide documentation that Toronto's outbreak was under control and to request that WHO remove the travel advisory' (National Advisory Committee, 2003, p. 202). Both provincial and federal governments in Canada criticized the WHO travel advisory as unwarranted in connection with Toronto (Heinzl and Chipello, 2003). Business and economic leaders in the Toronto community also complained that the travel advisory would further damage the tourism industry, which was already reeling from the SARS outbreak in Toronto (Heinzl and Chipello, 2003). As Health Canada's National Advisory Committee on SARS and Public Health later argued, 'the economic and social impact of such [travel] advisories can be devastating' and 'the effects of the travel advisories have been profound on the economies of targeted countries' (National Advisory Committee, 2003, pp. 37, 202). To the growing SARS problem, WHO now had to deal with Canadian anger and determination to have the travel advisory against Toronto lifted (Brown, 2003a).

Although WHO originally stated that its travel advisory against Toronto would be re-evaluated in three weeks (WHO, 2003p-1; Brown, 2003b), or twice the incubation period for SARS, WHO lifted its travel advisory against Toronto six days later, on 29 April (WHO, 2003s-1), after intense criticism and lobbying by the Canadian government (Brown, 2003c; Heinzl, 2003). WHO (2003s-1) cited four reasons for changing its mind about travel to the Canadian SARS 'hot zone': (1) the number of probable SARS cases in Toronto decreased in the week since the travel advisory was issued; (2) 20 days had passed since the last cases of SARS transmission in the community occurred; (3) no new confirmed cases of SARS exportation from Toronto had occurred; and (4) Canadian assurances that Canada would implement the pro-active passenger screening measures at airports recommended by WHO on 27 March. The WHO about-face on the Toronto travel advisory raised questions about whether politics played any role in the issuance and removal of the advisory (Frank, 2003), and such questions could only make WHO's job of controlling the worsening global SARS outbreak more difficult in the near future.

The third major reason why April witnessed a deepening of the SARS crisis was the behavior of China. As indicated earlier, March 2003 ended with mixed signals from China about the SARS outbreak. On the one hand, China promised to participate more actively in the WHO-led global campaign to control SARS. On the other hand, China was still behaving in ways that suggested it was not being entirely forthright about what was happening within its territory, as illustrated by the fact that the WHO team in Beijing had not been permitted, at the end of March, to visit Guangdong Province.

A pattern of ostensibly increasing Chinese cooperation appeared at the beginning of April 2003. On 1 April, the spokesman for the Chinese Foreign Ministry stated that '[t]he Chinese government has not covered up. There is no need. We have nothing to hide' (Wonacott, McKay, and Hamilton, 2003). On the same day that the WHO (2003b-1) issued its travel advisories against Hong Kong and Guangdong Province (2 April), China provided new data on the outbreak in Guangdong Province to cover the month of March. This new data pushed China's number of SARS cases to 1153, with 40 deaths, as of 31 March (WHO, 2003b-1). In addition to releasing new data on SARS in Guangdong Province, China approved the WHO team's visit to Guangdong to investigate the SARS outbreak there (WHO, 2003b-1). On 3 April, the Chinese Minister of Health announced on television that Beijing had only 12 cases of SARS and that the outbreak in China was under control (Cohen, Naik, and Pottinger, 2003). The same day China published a booklet entitled 'SARS is Nothing to Be Afraid Of' (Hiatt, 2003). On 4 April, China began submitting daily electronic reports to WHO on the SARS outbreak in its territory (WHO, 2003c-1).

Also on 4 April, the head of China's Center for Disease Control publicly apologized 'for failing to inform the public about a sometime fatal respiratory illness that has infected more than 2,000 people worldwide,' a statement that 'was unprecedented for a government that almost never acknowledges mistakes' (Pomfret, 2003g). The statement also contradicted earlier comments of Chinese government officials, such as the Minister of Health's statements on 3 April, that China had handled the outbreak properly (Pomfret, 2003g). WHO (2003d-1) praised China's decisions to put in place a system of alert and response for detection and reporting of all emerging and epidemic-prone diseases and to hold daily press conferences.

Events soon proved these Chinese moves toward cooperation and contrition to be duplicitous. The report of the WHO team that investigated the SARS outbreak in Guangdong Province praised the response of the provincial authorities but warned that other areas of China, such as Beijing, seemed much less prepared should SARS spread more widely in China (WHO, 2003f-1). On 7 April, China was reporting that Beijing had only 19 SARS cases (Pottinger and Hutzler, 2003) and four SARS-related deaths (WHO, 2003d-1). Doubts about this report from Beijing surfaced prominently when a staff member of the International Labour Organization (ILO), in Beijing for an ILO meeting, died of SARS in Beijing on 6 April (Pomfret, 2003h). WHO (2003d-1) noted on 7 April: 'At present it is unclear how the staff member contracted SARS. He had travelled to Beijing via Thailand, where no local transmission has been reported.' To explain the death of the ILO staff member, either the SARS situation in Thailand or Beijing had to be worse than was being reported to WHO. Although the Chinese Ministry of Health argued that the ILO staff member contracted SARS on a flight from Bangkok to Beijing (thus pointing the finger at Thailand as the source of the SARS infection), Chinese health officials did not try to track down other passengers on the same flight to check for other possible SARS infections (Hutzler, 2003a).

WHO's concerns about a SARS outbreak in Beijing intensified. On 9 April, news broke that a prominent Chinese doctor and Communist Party member, Jiang Yanyong, publicly accused the Chinese government of covering up the extent of the SARS outbreak in Beijing (Pomfret, 2003i). He argued that the actual number of SARS cases in Beijing was several times higher than what the government was reporting and that he and his colleagues were incredulous to hear the Chinese health minister saying on television (on 3 April) that the outbreak was under control (Pomfret, 2003i). Although Jiang originally sent his accusations against the government by e-mail to China Central Broadcasting and Phoenix Television based in Hong Kong, Jiang's bombshell made its impact after *Time Magazine* posted Jiang's e-mail on its web site, after which '*Time*'s report and a large number of other articles from the Western press were translated and sent to e-mail boxes all over China' (Pomfret, 2003r).

On 10 April, WHO asked the Chinese government if it could investigate the outbreak in Beijing to evaluate the validity of reports that the Beijing outbreak was much larger than China was reporting (Hutzler, 2003a). Henk Bekedam, head of WHO's office in Beijing, said on 10 April that '[t]here are various rumors right now, and we're not getting clear answers' (Pomfret, 2003i). On 11 April, WHO (2003g-1) diplomatically reported that '[p]articular concern centres on the situation in Beijing. Yesterday, WHO deepened discussions with Beijing health authorities, particularly concerning the efficiency of systems for case reporting and contact tracing.'

WHO (2003h-1) reported on 12 April that the Beijing Health Bureau invited a WHO team to visit health facilities in the city and to review generally the SARS outbreak in Beijing. On 14 April, the *Wall Street Journal* reported that Chinese officials were 'only slowly granting access' to the WHO investigating team, 'raising concerns about whether further outbreaks of the flu-like illness can be controlled worldwide without the full cooperation of China' (*Wall Street Journal*, 2003a). Also on 14 April, WHO (2003i-1) noted that authorities in Beijing 'have not granted WHO experts permission to visit military hospitals, which have been the focus of numerous rumors.'

Both news reports and WHO statements contained information on 15 April that China's government was beginning to understand the gravity of the concerns connected to the SARS outbreak in Beijing specifically and China generally. The *Wall Street Journal* reported on 15 April that 'China's government, publicly acknowledging that the spread of SARS poses serious risks for the country, is sounding its most urgent note yet about the pneumonia, as the number of new infections rose sharply' (Hutzler, 2003b). Chinese Premier Wen Jiabao warned that SARS could affect China's economy, international image, and social stability (Pomfret, 2003j). In keeping with this sense of heightened urgency coming from the Chinese government, WHO (2003j-1) announced on 15 April that '[t]he WHO team of experts in Beijing was today granted permission to visit military hospitals' and described this decision as 'a welcome indication of China's willingness to come to terms with the SARS outbreak on the mainland.'

Subsequent events revealed, however, that the new commitment and cooperative spirit shown by the Chinese government was, yet again, a charade. The *Washington Post* reported on 16 April that Chinese physicians accused government officials of 'significantly underreporting both the incidence of severe acute respiratory syndrome in China's capital and the role Beijing plays as a new source of the disease's spread' (Pomfret, 2003k). The *Washington Post* added that the reason for the cover-up in Beijing was fear that WHO would issue travel advisories against Beijing, as it had for Hong Kong and Guangdong Province, if the true number of SARS cases in the city were reported (Pomfret, 2003k). The WHO team in Beijing indicated that it was still not receiving full information from Beijing government officials about the SARS situation (Pomfret, 2003k). Unofficial information provided by local doctors about China's official underreporting of SARS cases around the country also began to increase (Jakes, 2003), bolstering the view that China was continuing to try to cover up the epidemic.

By this point in the SARS outbreak, China's role in the epidemic had become clear; and, as the epicenter of the SARS outbreak, WHO and others working on the global SARS effort knew that effective Chinese action on SARS was critical to containing this new disease's global potential. Yet, by 15 April, repeated attempts to hide the full scale of the outbreak marred China's cooperation in the global campaign against SARS. China's behavior was deepening the SARS crisis because the key to containing the global outbreak of SARS was controlling SARS-CoV in China. Foreign reporters in China were also starting to chastise WHO for not confronting China's cover-up (Cohen, Naik, and Pottinger, 2003). How this situation unfolded would shape the fight against SARS and its prospects for success.

In an unprecedented move, WHO went on the offensive against China. On 16 April, the *Washington Post* reported the following:

> The World Health Organization said today that China is underreporting cases of the SARS virus and maintains secret military files that make it impossible to control and monitor the spread of the disease in the Chinese capital. WHO researchers, speaking in unusually blunt language, said at a news conference that the government has misled the public about the spread of severe acute respiratory syndrome, or SARS. Officials said the number of patients infected with the virus in Beijing could be 200, more than five times what the government has acknowledged. 'We have very clearly said you have an international community over here that does not trust your figures,' said Henk Bekedam, head of the office of the World Health Organization in Beijing. (Pomfret, 2003l)

WHO estimated that Beijing had as many as 200 SARS cases even though government officials had only reported 37 cases (WHO, 2003m-1; Pomfret, 2003m). The *Wall Street Journal* referred to these WHO statements as the delivery of 'a humiliating public rebuke to Beijing officials for downplaying the extent of the disease' (Pottinger, 2003c).

At its press conference, WHO's criticism extended beyond the Beijing situation because WHO stated that it had not 'received sufficient information to determine the scale of the outbreak in China, the epicenter of the mysterious new disease' (Wonacott, Lawrence, and Pottinger, 2003). Further, WHO even expressed concern about China's overall approach to public health. WHO's Henk Bekedam indicated that 'he was concerned that unless China allocated more money for public health, poor people would not be able to pay for treatment if they contract SARS. "We do believe that the government has not invested in health in the last 30 years," he said. "The government has left it to the people to pay for health care and who among the poor will be able to afford treatment?"' (Pomfret, 2003l).

Typically, WHO refrains from publicly criticizing its member states because such criticism puts the intergovernmental organization in a difficult position in its work with member governments. WHO's public criticism of the Chinese government represented a radical break with the traditional diplomacy that characterizes relations between the Organization and member states. Such a radical move by WHO underscores the urgency with which it viewed the deepening SARS crisis. The sweeping nature of the criticism from WHO, which involved the Beijing situation, the outbreak in China generally, and the Chinese government's neglect of public health, was also breathtaking. These actions by WHO suggest that the Organization concluded that 'business as usual' with the Chinese government was not going to provide a sufficiently robust response to bring SARS under control in China and, thus, reduce the threat SARS in China would pose to other countries. As with the issuance of the travel advisories earlier in the month, WHO's public criticism of China was a bold act in its effort to lead the global campaign against SARS.

WHO's boldness was rewarded with a transformation of Chinese policy on SARS. But this transformation did not occur without the help of one final, embarrassing incident for the Chinese government. On 16 April, Chinese officials allowed the WHO's experts to begin visiting military and other hospitals in the Beijing area (WHO, 2003l-1). As later reported in *Time*, 'hospital officials removed dozens of SARS patients from their isolation wards and transferred them to locations where they could not be observed by the inspectors' (Jakes, 2003). On 18 April, *Time* published an exposé of the Chinese government's attempts to hoodwink WHO personnel (Jakes, 2003). With information provided by doctors and medical staff at hospitals subject to WHO visits, *Time* revealed a large-scale effort to hide the size of the SARS outbreak in Beijing from WHO through the transfer of dozens of SARS patients out of hospitals to facilities not visited by WHO (Jakes, 2003). 'These actions,' observed the *Washington Post*, '...mark the most egregious in a series of steps taken by the Chinese government to cover up the extent of the epidemic' (Pomfret, 2003n).

On 18 April, the leaders of China's Communist Party 'declared a nationwide war on the SARS virus and ordered officials to stop covering up the extent of the epidemic that is spreading throughout China' (Pomfret, 2003m). According to WHO (2003m-1), China's Communist Party leaders demanded accurate, timely, and honest reporting of SARS cases, called SARS a serious threat to the country's reforms, development, and stability, and warned that Party and government officials would be held accountable for the SARS situation in their respective jurisdictions.

On 20 April, the Communist Party removed the Minister of Health and mayor of Beijing from their Party posts for their role in covering up the SARS epidemic in China (Pomfret, 2003o). The Chinese government also increased, on 20 April, the number of confirmed SARS cases in Beijing from 37 to 346, 'a tacit acknowledgement that it had previously lied about the toll' (Pomfret, 2003o). On 21 April, China reported another 109 SARS cases in Beijing (WHO, 2003o-1); and the Secretary of Beijing's Communist Party issued an apology for the mishandling of the epidemic (Pomfret, 2003p). Also on 21 April, the Chinese government cancelled the traditional week-long May Day holiday to prevent hundreds of thousands of people from traveling throughout the country and contributing to the spread of SARS (WHO, 2003o-1; Pomfret, 2003p). Toward the end of April, China also closed movie theaters, discos, Internet bars, public libraries, and churches; quarantined thousands of people and dozens of hospitals; and fired two more high-ranking officials for failing to handle SARS appropriately (Pomfret, 2003q). These, and subsequent actions by the Chinese government, demonstrated that China had finally stopped trying to cover up the SARS epidemic and had moved to mount a vigorous nation-wide response to SARS, working closely with WHO and other elements of the global SARS effort.

As noted earlier, WHO (2003p-1) issued travel advisories against Beijing and Shanxi Province on 23 April because of the magnitude of the outbreaks in those areas, the extent of local chains of transmission, and evidence that travelers were becoming infected while in those areas and then exporting the disease elsewhere. China was now subject to four WHO travel advisories – for Hong Kong, Guangdong Province, Beijing, and Shanxi Province – an indication of the overall seriousness of the SARS problem in China, the danger of local transmission, and the threat China's SARS situation posed for international travel and the public health in other countries.

With improved reporting from the Chinese government, WHO noted at the end of April 2003 that SARS cases had been reported in 21 of China's 31 provinces (WHO, 2003s-1) and that China's 3460 probable SARS cases accounted for more cases than the rest of the world combined (WHO, 2003t-1). Although the Chinese government appeared to have changed its behavior significantly by the end of April, precious time and opportunities to bring China's SARS outbreak under control had been lost in April. Whether WHO's boldness in challenging China's behavior, and China's subsequent policy reversal, would allow the global campaign to contain the SARS epicenter in China remained worryingly unclear as April 2003 came to a close.

May 2003: Turning the corner

During May 2003, the global SARS outbreak continued to grow. On 1 May, WHO (2003u-1) reported a cumulative total of 5865 probable SARS cases with 391 deaths involving 27 countries. On 29 May, WHO (2003m-2) reported a cumulative total of 8295 cases with 750 deaths from 28 countries. Unlike the growth of the epidemic in April, the May increase in SARS cases and deaths did not represent a deepening of the SARS crisis. In fact, developments during the course of May indicated that the global effort to bring SARS under control was beginning to turn the corner on bringing the outbreak under control. WHO's Mike Ryan captured the mood in mid-May when he said that the message to take away from the progress achieved to date was 'one of celebration that the measures are working, but also a call to action because we've got a lot more to do yet before we end this problem' (Stein, 2003h).

The most visible signs of progress came from most of the original SARS 'hot zones' – Guangdong Province, Hong Kong, Singapore, and Vietnam. Each of these SARS-affected areas experienced significant progress from late April until the end of May in handling their SARS outbreaks. WHO announced on 28 April that Vietnam had become the first country to succeed in containing the SARS epidemic when Vietnam detected no new SARS cases for 20 days (WHO, 2003r-1; Nakashima, 2003a).

Singapore's success in controlling its outbreak during May was evident when WHO (2003n-2) removed Singapore on 31 May from the list of areas with recent local transmission of SARS. Singapore was initially scheduled to be removed from the list of SARS-affected areas on 11 May; but, on that date, Singapore reported a new case of SARS to WHO, an indication of Singapore's commitment to open reporting and cooperation with WHO (WHO, 2003n-2).

Progress was also apparent in connection with three of the hottest 'hot zones' – Hong Kong, Guangdong Province, and Toronto. As noted above, WHO lifted the travel advisories for Toronto on 30 April. On 14 May, WHO (2003b-2) dropped Toronto from its list of areas experiencing local SARS transmission. WHO (2003i-2) lifted the advisories for Hong Kong and Guangdong Province on 23 May because 'the situation in these areas has now improved significantly.' The health authorities in Hong Kong and Guangdong Province succeeded during May in reducing the number of new cases and the extent of local transmission and in preventing exported cases (WHO, 2003i-2).

The examples of Vietnam, Singapore, Toronto, Hong Kong, and Guangdong Province underscored WHO's comments in its 13 May SARS update that '[e]xperiences in a growing number of countries indicate that the disease can be contained, thus supporting WHO's overall objective: to prevent SARS from becoming widely established as another new disease in humans' (WHO, 2003a-2). Supporting the approach being taken against SARS was the failure of new 'hot zones' to develop despite the SARS virus spreading to 28 countries by the end of May. Many countries reported a small number of cases of SARS; but, except for one country (Taiwan), these cases did not develop into epidemics within those countries because of appropriate surveillance and response activities implemented by public health officials. WHO noted, for example, that only one case of SARS transmission had occurred on European soil during the outbreak (Richburg, 2003).

The progress made in the SARS 'hot zones' and the success in keeping SARS under control in most countries into which the SARS virus was imported occurred, by and large, without the global SARS campaign gaining any new technological weapons developed from scientific research or benefiting directly from breakthroughs in scientific knowledge about SARS. In May 2003, WHO revised its SARS case definition 'to take into account the appropriate use of results from laboratory tests'; but WHO continued to warn against the inappropriate use of diagnostic tests in connection with dealing with suspected SARS cases because all such available tests have weaknesses (WHO, 2003u-1).

The global SARS efforts witnessed the development of more scientific and epidemiological knowledge about SARS, including studies on the environmental survivability of SARS-CoV (WHO, 2003w-1; WHO, 2003c-2), the overall case fatality rate (WHO, 2003x-1), the incubation period of SARS-CoV (WHO, 2003x-1), risk of SARS transmission during air travel (WHO, 2003e-2; WHO, 2003h-2), and the presence of SARS-CoV in wild animals in southern China (WHO, 2003j-2). Experts discussed many of these topics at the first global consultation on SARS epidemiology held at WHO headquarters in Geneva on 16–17 May (WHO, 2003d-2). These scientific endeavors did not, however, change WHO's recommended surveillance and response approaches to SARS cases, including 'the earliest possible isolation of all suspect and probable cases of SARS' (WHO, 2003x-1).

Although significant progress was seen in the original SARS 'hot zones' and in new countries of SARS importation, the global SARS effort continued to face difficult challenges in May 2003. Foremost among these challenges was the continuing struggle to contain SARS in China. As WHO (2003u-1) stated on 1 May, '[t]he next few months will prove crucial in the attempt to contain SARS worldwide, which now greatly depends on whether the disease can be controlled in China.' Evidence of the difficulty of this task can be found in the travel advisories WHO issued against the following Chinese provinces during May 2003: Tianjin, Inner Mongolia, and Hebei (WHO, 2003y-1; WHO, 2003d-2). Thus, at the end of May, four Chinese provinces and Beijing were subject to WHO advisories recommending that non-essential travel to these areas be postponed. These advisories meant that WHO had concluded that the number of new cases of SARS, extent of local transmission, and threat of SARS exportation remained significant in these areas.

Questions remained, and cropped up, about Chinese-generated data during May 2003, as illustrated by the puzzlement WHO officials expressed at the end of May concerning China's reports of very low numbers of new cases and deaths related to SARS (Chen *et al.*, 2003). In addition, tensions between China and WHO flared at the end of May when the Deputy Minister of Health, Gao Qiang, argued at a news conference on 30 May that the Chinese government had not concealed the outbreak and claimed that its February notifications to WHO alerted the world to the problem (Cherney and Chang, 2003). According to journalist Laurie Garret (2003), WHO 'went ballistic' and sternly warned China that '[i]f you're going to try and tell us that you were not lying before, ... we are going to have to pull our office out of Beijing. We can't work with you anymore.' WHO's response prompted Gao to reappear a few days later to recant his 30 May claims, ending what could have been a much more serious crisis. Despite these questions and tension, neither WHO nor news reports indicated that China's government was backtracking on its commitment to fight SARS vigorously. As the *Wall Street Journal* put it, 'China is as good at fighting SARS as at hiding it' (Chen, 2003).

China, now more forcefully assisted by WHO and other international partners, faced not only the epidemiological challenge of SARS but also the high level of distrust and anxiety China's attempt to cover up the epidemic had caused in the Chinese population. China's more rigorous response to containing the epidemic, which including improved surveillance activities, heightened infection control procedures in health care facilities dealing with SARS cases, closing schools, and instituting large-scale quarantines, began to show some positive, if tentative, effects by mid-May.

The *Wall Street Journal* reported on 13 May the declining number of daily cases China was notifying but quoted epidemiologists as arguing that it was too soon to read much into such declines (Chang, 2003a). Interestingly, on the same day, China's leaders again demanded that government officials provide full and immediate data on the outbreak (Pomfret, 2003s). Although WHO still had concerns about the lack of full information from China's military, it 'praised China for beginning to take the disease seriously but cautioned that the epidemic had not begun to fade' (Pomfret, 2003s; Chang, 2003b).

In addition to the ongoing struggle in China, the global SARS effort had to deal with some new problems in May 2003. WHO added Mongolia (WHO, 2003u-1) and the Philippines (WHO, 2003x-1) to the list of areas experiencing recent local transmission of SARS in early May, suggesting that SARS was making inroads into two countries not previously considered problem areas. Fortunately, WHO removed both Mongolia and the Philippines from its list of SARS-affected areas later in the month, demonstrating that these countries had brought local transmission of SARS under control (WHO, 2003z-1; WHO, 2003f-2).

The most troubling new problem to arise in May was the SARS outbreak in Taiwan. Although Taiwan had been on WHO's initial list of SARS-affected areas in late March, the epidemic in Taiwan worsened in late April and early May. On 2 May, the *Wall Street Journal* observed that '[o]utside of mainland China, Taiwan's SARS outbreak is now the fastest moving in all of Asia' (Regalado and Dean, 2003). WHO (2003v-1) reported on 3 May that '[t]he spread of SARS in Taiwan has accelerated considerably during the past week.' With the permission of China, a WHO team began to provide assistance to Taiwan in early May as the Taiwanese outbreak grew (WHO, 2003v-1). On 8 May, WHO issued a travel advisory against Taipei (WHO, 2003y-1); and, on 21 May, WHO extended the advisory to cover all of Taiwan, indicating that WHO believed that the magnitude of the outbreak in Taiwan, the extent of local transmission on the island, and the potential for exportation of

SARS were significantly high for the entire territory of Taiwan (WHO, 2003g-2).

Vigorous action by the Taiwanese authorities, assisted by WHO, began to show results even before the month of May ended. On 28 May, WHO (2003l-2) reported that the latest notification of new cases from Taiwan marked 'the continuation of a downward trend that became apparent earlier in the week' and opined that Taiwan was 'now much closer to bringing SARS under control.' The progress made in the Taiwanese SARS outbreak continued to confirm the effectiveness of the surveillance and response approaches the global SARS campaign had developed, refined, and implemented in many different jurisdictions.

By the end of May 2003, the ongoing SARS outbreaks in China and Taiwan were more than sufficient to keep the global SARS campaign from becoming complacent about the threat SARS posed. The re-emergence of local transmission of SARS in Toronto at the end of May highlighted the continuing danger SARS-CoV posed and the need for vigilance on the part of public health officials and health care facilities (WHO, 2003k-2; Brown, 2003d). Infectious disease experts in the United States warned of resurgence of SARS in the winter months of late 2003 and early 2004 (Connolly, 2003). Fears remained about SARS spreading to 'the less-developed parts of Asia and Africa, which have far less effective health systems to identify and isolate cases, and vast populations especially vulnerable to new infections because of AIDS' (Stein, 2003g; Stein, 2003i).

The global SARS campaign received a significant boost at the annual World Health Assembly at the end of May 2003. The World Health Assembly – WHO's highest policy-making body – approved two resolutions that supported WHO's leadership on, and actions taken during, the SARS outbreak. In the resolution on SARS, the World Health Assembly described SARS as 'the first severe infectious disease to emerge in the twenty-first century' and recognized that SARS 'poses a serious threat to global health security, the livelihood of populations, the functioning of health systems, and the stability and growth of economies' (World Health Assembly, 2003a). The World Health Assembly acknowledged the need for intensive and urgent international collaboration and noted WHO's crucial role in leading the world-wide campaign to control and contain SARS. The SARS resolution also urged WHO member states to implement many of the lessons learned in the SARS effort, such as the importance of reporting cases promptly and transparently to WHO.

The resolution on the revision of the International Health Regulations (IHR) indicated that the SARS experience had confirmed the inadequacy of the existing IHR, urged WHO member states to support the IHR revision process, and requested the WHO Director-General to continue to use non-governmental sources of information as part of global surveillance activities, to issue global health alerts about the presence of a public health threat that may constitute a serious threat to neighboring countries or to international health, and to collaborate with governments in assessing the severity of public health threats and the adequacy of response measures (World Health Assembly, 2003b). The IHR resolution paved the way for the actions taken and lessons learned in the SARS outbreak to form part of the governance responses to future infectious disease threats – a clear indication that the SARS outbreak was becoming more than a public health crisis and was beginning to serve as a model for future global public health policy.

June 2003: 'Stopped dead in its tracks'

June 2003 opened with WHO recognizing further progress against SARS, indicating that the momentum generated in May continued strongly. On 4 June, WHO reported that no deaths from SARS had been reported, the first time since 28 March that no country reported any SARS-related fatalities (WHO, 2003o-2; Stein, 2003j). WHO (2003o-2) commented that, '[w]ith outbreaks in all the initial "hot zones" either contained or coming under control, SARS is clearly in decline, indicating that recommended control measures are effective when combined with political commitment and determination.'

The progress was particularly evident with respect to China, the SARS epicenter. Between 6 June and 9 June, China reported only one probable new case of SARS (WHO 2003p-2). WHO officials began a visit to China on 10 June 'to learn which measures taken by China have so rapidly brought the country's SARS outbreak – the largest in the world – under control' (WHO, 2003q-2). More tangible evidence of China's progress against SARS came on 13 June when WHO lifted its travel advisories against the Chinese provinces of Hebei, Inner Mongolia, Shanxi, and Tianjin and removed Guangdong, Hebei, Hubei, Inner Mongolia, Jilin, Jiangsu, Shaanxi, Shanxi, and Tianjin from the list of areas with recent local transmission (WHO, 2003s-2). These moves left Beijing as the last area in China on the list of areas with local SARS transmission and subject to a WHO travel advisory, and WHO removed Beijing from the local-transmission list and lifted this advisory on 24 June (WHO, 2003w-2). The progress made in China against SARS in May and June was nothing short of stunning.

Further evidence that SARS was in retreat came when WHO removed, on 23 June, Hong Kong – one of the original SARS 'hot zones' – from the list of areas experiencing local transmission (WHO, 2003v-2). By the end of June 2003, no countries remained subject to a WHO travel advisory and only Toronto and Taiwan remained on the list of areas experiencing local transmission of SARS. WHO removed Toronto from this list on July 2 (WHO, 2003z-2), and Taiwan on 5 July (WHO, 2003a-3).

On 17 June, WHO Director-General Gro Harlem Brundtland told the first global conference on SARS in Kuala Lumpur, Malaysia that, on the eve of the outbreak's hundredth day, the world, in the face of 'a new disease, striking a globalized society,' has 'seen unprecedented international solidarity against a shared microbial threat of unknown dimensions' (Brundtland, 2003). She argued that the remarkable speed and sweep of the achievements of the global SARS efforts meant that 'we have seen SARS stopped dead in its tracks in some of the worst affected areas' (Brundtland, 2003). On 27 June, WHO declared that the world should be free of human SARS cases in two or three weeks (Reuters, 2003).

The effective end of the SARS outbreak in all countries during June 2003 meant that WHO began switching gears on SARS. As WHO (2003x-2) observed on 30 June, '[a]s no new cases of SARS have been reported anywhere in the world since 15 June, WHO is moving from an emergency response to a research-based agenda aimed at protecting the world against any future resurgence of SARS.' During June, as the SARS outbreaks in all countries were brought under control, WHO repeatedly warned that political and public health vigilance continued to be vital against SARS (WHO, 2003o-2; WHO, 2003r-2; WHO, 2003t-2; WHO, 2003a-3). WHO (2003t-2) argued on 18 June that '[a]s long as a single case of SARS exists or is suspected anywhere in the world, and as long as fundamental questions about the origins of the virus remain unanswered, all countries need to remain on guard.' On 5 July, WHO (2003a-3) warned that 'SARS will continue to menace the global public health system.'

Stopping SARS 'dead in its tracks' less than four months after the appearance of this new virus and respiratory disease in the globalized world of the early twenty-first century will undoubtedly rank as one of the great success stories in the history of global public health efforts on infectious diseases, and the greatest achievement in this realm since the eradication of smallpox in the late 1970s. What this chapter's brief history of the SARS outbreak does not adequately communicate, however, is the landmark significance of the SARS outbreak to governance of infectious diseases. The next two chapters explore this historic feature of the global SARS outbreak of 2002–03.

6
China Confronts Public Health's 'New World Order'

How the victory was won

The successful handling of the SARS outbreak by WHO's global campaign was a significant victory for public health. The success of the SARS effort stands in marked contrast to a parade of worsening infectious disease problems identified in the 1990s and early 2000s under the moniker of 'emerging and re-emerging infectious diseases.' Thinking about why the SARS campaign achieved stunning results does not lead analysis into biomedical technologies, such as vaccines, which have contributed greatly to improvements in prevention, control, and eradication of other pathogenic threats, such as smallpox. The WHO-led global campaign contained SARS without having access to adequate diagnostic technologies, effective anti-viral therapies, or a vaccine. The public health instruments at the forefront of the SARS battle were surveillance, isolation, and quarantine, which were the main tools of infectious disease control in the historical era before the development of the arsenal of vaccines and antibiotics.

How, then, did a public health effort, armed only with essentially nineteenth-century public health instruments, succeed in stopping a contagious pathogen in twenty-first century, globalized conditions dead in its tracks within four months of the epidemic's first recognition? Answering this question involves understanding the governance context in which the SARS effort took place. Chapter 4 described the trends in governance with respect to infectious diseases that developed during the 1990s and early 2000s. A shift from Westphalian public health governance to a post-Westphalian governance framework is apparent in these trends; but, prior to SARS, the shift was still nascent or, as was the case with HIV/AIDS, tapped at a point when an epidemic was already out of control. As the first severe infectious disease to emerge in the twenty-first century, SARS represented a critical test of post-Westphalian public health governance. Understanding how the SARS victory was won requires examining how post-Westphalian public health governance – in both conception and implementation – passed the test posed by the SARS outbreak.

China: Epidemiological and governance epicenter

As Chapter 5 demonstrated, public health experts recognized that China represented the epidemiological epicenter of the SARS outbreak. WHO repeatedly argued that SARS would not be controlled globally unless China controlled SARS domestically. Therefore, China's behavior was critical to the functioning of post-Westphalian governance for infectious diseases. China was the governance epicenter because of the task it had in dealing with the largest SARS outbreak within its borders and how the Chinese management of this task interfaced with global SARS efforts. China provides the best case study for analyzing the governance shift in infectious disease control because China acted Westphalian in a post-Westphalian world.

For this reason, China's response to SARS proved a miscalculation of historic proportions. The miscalculation involves not only the damage China suffered to its economy but also China's failure to grasp the post-Westphalian context of infectious disease governance. The saga of the SARS outbreak in China tells the story of the humbling of the sovereignty of a rising great power. The humbling of Chinese sovereignty occurred in both traditional public health areas, such as surveillance and response, and matters of political ideology. As a result of its response to SARS, China suffered extensive and withering scrutiny and criticism of its attitude toward public health, its health care system, and the political ideology underlying governance in that country.

China, SARS, and Westphalian public health

As Chapter 5 detailed, China's response to SARS divides into three stages. The first stage, which began in November 2002 and lasted until early February 2003, witnessed the Chinese government's attempt to suppress information about a severe outbreak of a mysterious respiratory disease in Guangdong Province. These attempts to suppress information did not succeed, as news of the outbreak leaked out through the Internet, e-mail, mobile phone text messaging, and the local Chinese media.

The second stage of China's response began in mid-February 2003 and lasted until 17 April 2003. In this stage, China acknowledged an outbreak but attempted to deny and cover up the extent of the epidemic. A pattern emerged during this stage: China would admit there was a problem, make moves to appear to be enhancing international cooperation, but, after each strategic retreat, try again to cover up the full extent of the SARS outbreak. This pattern continued through the Chinese attempt to hide SARS patients from WHO personnel visiting Beijing hospitals to assess the real level of infection in the capital. China also made various claims during this period, such as the outbreak in Guangdong Province had been contained by mid-February and had not spread to other parts of China, all of which eventually proved to be deliberate falsehoods promulgated by the Chinese government. As during the first stage of its response, China could not control the flow of information about the SARS problem from reaching the outside world; and this information destroyed the credibility of the official claims of the Chinese government and brought the entire Chinese governance system into disrepute.

The third stage of China's response began on 18 April 2003 when China's Communist Party finally called a halt to the systematic deception it had been orchestrating on SARS. From that date on, China increased the information it provided to WHO, improved its cooperation with WHO and other countries, and heightened the seriousness of its SARS control efforts. As Chapter 5 indicated, the results from this reversal of policy were impressive because China succeeded in bringing a very bad SARS epidemic within its borders under effective control within two months.

Stepping back from the detailed analysis of events provided in Chapter 5, one can see that the first two stages of China's response to SARS conform to the patterns of the Westphalian approach to infectious disease control. As analyzed in Chapter 3, the central concept of Westphalian governance is sovereignty. A state has supreme power over the people who live, and the events that transpire, within its territory. Under the Westphalian framework, such supreme power remains unfettered until the state consents to exercise its sovereignty in the manner prescribed by rules of international law. This dynamic applied equally to public health as to other areas of international relations – states disciplined their sovereignty over public health within their territories through rules of international law negotiated and accepted by them.

From the perspective of Westphalian public health, the first two stages of China's response to SARS were understandable. China was under no international legal obligation to report SARS cases to any state or international organization. The only set of international legal rules directly affecting surveillance for infectious diseases – the International Health Regulations (IHR) – did not include SARS on the list of diseases subject to the notification duties binding on WHO member states (IHR, 1969, Article 1). Similarly, China was under no international legal obligation to involve WHO in addressing the SARS problem within Chinese territory. China could utilize WHO in dealing with SARS, if it chose to do so, but remained in complete control over where WHO personnel could go and how WHO operated while in China. Demands to the contrary from WHO or any other state would represent intervention in China's domestic affairs and an affront to its sovereignty.

These observations challenge 'numerous comments from academics and politicians both here and abroad that China's apparent inaction is tantamount to dereliction of duty; i.e., that Beijing was obligated to take measures to prevent the spread of the disease and inform the international community of the danger posed by the virus' (Bishop, 2003). Many public health officials and political leaders have criticized the manner in which the Chinese government responded to the SARS outbreak. US Secretary of Health and Human Services Tommy Thompson argued, for example, that China's behavior cost lives in other countries (Pomfret, 2003o). Such comments and criticisms have raised the question of whether China's behavior created any responsibility for it under international law.

According to the draft Articles on Responsibility of States for International Wrongful Acts promulgated by the United Nations' International Law Commission, '[e]very internationally wrongful act of a State entails the international responsibility of that State' (International Law Commission, 2001, Article 1). An internationally wrongful act by a state occurs when a state's action or omission is attributable to that state under international law and constitutes a breach of an international legal obligation of the state (International Law Commission, 2001, Article 2). An act by a state 'does not constitute a breach of an international obligation unless the State is bound by the obligation in question at the time the act occurs' (International Law Commission, 2001, Article 13).

In order for China's reluctance to share epidemiological information on disease events in its territory under its control, or China's non-cooperative attitude toward WHO in the first two stages of its response to SARS, to be an internationally wrongful act, China would have to be in breach of some international legal obligation that it consented to obey and that was applicable at the time the SARS outbreak occurred.

As indicated earlier, China's international legal obligations under the IHR are to report outbreaks of cholera, plague, and yellow fever. China is under no other international legal obligation to report other disease events to WHO or other states.

In terms of treaty law, the WHO Constitution does not impose on member states any specific duty to control infectious diseases or to cooperate with the Organization on infectious disease problems. The only concrete duties WHO member states have agreed to undertake in accepting the WHO Constitution are to pay their financial assessments and submit certain general reports to WHO (WHO, 1948, Articles 7, 61–65).

Under customary international law, states are under no obligation unless a rule of custom is supported by general and consistent state practice and a sense on the part of states that such practice is legally binding on their behavior (*opinio juris*) (Brownlie, 1998, pp. 3–9). Finding general and consistent state practice on reporting infectious disease outbreaks would be a futile effort for two reasons. First, this aspect of international relations has, since 1851, been handled as a matter of treaty law not custom. Second, the failure of states to comply with their treaty obligation on disease reporting found in the IHR render impossible the discovery of state practice and *opinio juris* supporting infectious disease notification obligations as a matter of customary international law.

In the absence of an international legal obligation that applies to its actions directly on SARS, China's behavior cannot be considered legally wrongful under international legal principles of state responsibility. China's behavior made the public health threat posed by SARS worse; but, given the configuration of international law in place at the time of China's actions, China's exercise of its sovereignty does not appear to trigger state responsibility under international law. To pursue China's international legal responsibility under these principles, we have to leave the specific context of infectious disease control and make analogies to contexts regulated by international environmental law.

Eminent scholars of international law on environmental protection have argued that '[i]t is beyond serious argument that states are required by international law to take adequate steps to control and regulate sources of serious global environmental pollution or transboundary harm within their territory or subject to their jurisdiction' (Birnie and Boyle, 1992, p. 89). One could argue that, under the general concept expressed by this purported rule, international law obligates states to take adequate steps to control and regulate sources of serious global public health threats or transboundary public health harm within their territory or subject to their jurisdiction. Recognizing that much of international environmental law addresses threats to public health (Fidler, 2001b, p. 10048) strengthens the connection between the rule of international environmental law and cross-border threats from infectious diseases.

Two problems, however, undermine this argument by analogy to international environmental law. First, scholars have, in fact, challenged the assertion that international law, without question, requires states to control and regulate sources of global environmental pollution and transboundary harm within their territories or under their jurisdiction. This rule is presented as a rule of customary international law, and customary international law embodies the unwritten, common law rules for state interaction in anarchy. As indicated above, rules of customary international law form when states recognize as legally binding principles drawn from general and consistent state practice on a particular issue.

As scholars of international environmental law have observed, global and transboundary pollution by states is the norm not the exception, meaning that there is not general and consistent state practice that states act to reduce global and transboundary environmental harm (Bodansky, 1995, pp. 110–11; Schacter, 1991, pp. 462–3). The repeated resort to treaty law as a way to deal with global and transboundary environmental harm caused by state activities within their borders further illustrates the weakness of the purported rule of customary international law.

Second, the customary principle of responsibility to prevent, reduce, and control global or transboundary environmental harm translates awkwardly into the infectious disease context. To begin, one would search in vain for general and consistent state practice with respect to infectious disease control supporting a customary rule that states have to take adequate steps to control and regulate sources of serious global public health threats or transboundary harm within their territory or subject to their jurisdiction. As the historical experience of the IHR illustrates, states have addressed international infectious disease control through treaty law not customary international law. Again, the routine violation of the IHR by WHO member states during its lifetime underscores the futility of trying to use customary international law to find a general duty on infectious diseases applicable to China in the context of SARS.

Another reason why the analogy to international environmental law transfers badly to the infectious disease situation involves the breach element of international law on state responsibility. Even if a principle of international law existed requiring all states to address sources of global or transboundary infectious disease harm within their territories, what would constitute a breach of this obligation? Would China's efforts to contain the initial outbreak in Guangdong Province from November 2002 and February 2003 represent a breach, even though it did take some steps (albeit in secret) to control the infectious disease problem? Is the standard for breach strict liability, gross negligence, or just negligence?

Perhaps China's failure to notify WHO and other states about the true extent of the outbreak within its territory constitutes the breach of a general customary duty to deal with infectious disease problems inside its territory. But we have come full circle analytically because, as the long history of the classical international legal regime on infectious diseases demonstrates, states have dealt with surveillance for purposes of international control of infectious diseases through treaty law not customary international law. And, at the time of the SARS outbreak, China's treaty commitments on infectious diseases did not involve obligations to report SARS cases. Thus, failure to report SARS information openly, transparently, and in a timely way constituted no violation of applicable international law. Attempts to catch China in violation of international legal principles developed for Westphalian public health resembles grasping for straws in the wind.

Another feature of China's response to SARS that resonates with the Westphalian model is China's status as a rising great power in the international system. As illustrated in Chapter 3, Westphalian public health functioned under the direction of the world's great powers. China's increasing political and economic importance in international relations provides evidence of China's power and position in world politics. The United States views, for example, China as a strategic competitor. China's accession to the World Trade Organization in 2001 solidified that nation's significance to world trade. In 2002, China surpassed the United States as the world's leading destination for foreign direct investment. China is also considered the critical player in managing the stand-off that has developed over North Korea's attempts to develop nuclear weapons.

Under Westphalian public health, China's status as a rising great power should have given China a preferential role in shaping responses to infectious disease problems. Similarly, other states and international organizations should defer to the great power's exercise of its sovereignty over matters taking place in its territory. The interests of the great powers in infectious disease control in the Westphalian template were two-fold: (1) to prevent and reduce disease importation from weaker, poorer countries; and (2) to minimize the burden public health measures impose on international trade. Westphalian public health governance did not entail scrutiny of public health policy and practices within the territory of the great powers. The first two stages of China's response to SARS conformed to the Westphalian dynamic because China behaved in ways that indicated it believed the SARS problem in its territory was exclusively its sovereign concern.

Analysis of the traditional rules of international law on, and political dynamics of, infectious disease control support the argument that China's initial response to SARS follows the tenets of Westphalian public health. This argument does not claim that China responded to SARS by saying 'let's act Westphalian.' In fact, the reasons why China behaved in the way it did are more complex than simple analytical concepts. For example, the nature of Communist Party rule in China forms part of the story of China's actions in the face of SARS. But this factor again brings back the importance of the Westphalian template, under which the nature of a state's government and ideology are not diplomatic issues. Westphalian governance concepts, particularly the principle of non-intervention in the domestic affairs of other states, steer diplomacy away from the nature of a country's domestic political and economic structures toward management of the mechanistic interactions of states in their anarchical condition.

This extended discussion of international law and politics on infectious diseases underscores the main point of this section: The first two stages of China's response to SARS conform to the Westphalian template for public health governance. These observations do not mean that China's response to SARS was prudent merely because it conformed to Westphalian patterns. Nothing in the Westphalian model prevented China from responding more openly and cooperatively, as other nations did. More broadly, the absence of specific international legal obligations in the WHO Constitution on infectious diseases does not prevent WHO member states from working with WHO to prevent and control infectious disease problems in their territories. Most member states cooperate with WHO on public health problems in the absence of direct international legal obligations to do so.

The main point of connecting China's behavior to the Westphalian approach to public health is that this approach did not demand more from China with respect to SARS. Westphalian public health left China's sovereignty unfettered and to be exercised, for better or worse, as China's government saw fit. Westphalian public health is based on a governance model developed originally through nineteenth-century diplomacy on infectious diseases. The crisis in emerging and re-emerging infectious diseases had already begun to call this governance model into question prior to SARS, and the SARS outbreak further revealed the mistake of trying to address twenty-first century infectious disease threats through a nineteenth-century governance framework.

Westphalian sovereignty v. global health governance

The best way to analyze the mistakes China made in connection with SARS is to examine the outcome of the confrontation between China's response to SARS, which resonates with the traditional Westphalian approach, and the emerging mechanics and objectives of post-Westphalian public health, namely global health governance and global public goods for health. This section focuses on China's experience with SARS in light of global health governance, and the subsequent section explores China's behavior with respect to the concept of global public goods for health.

In many ways, China exercised its sovereignty during the SARS outbreak in the same way that states often behaved with respect to past disease outbreaks. States have frequently failed to notify WHO and other states about outbreaks in their territories, even when international law (e.g., IHR) required such notifications. Even when news of outbreaks did reach the outside world, states often did not provide accurate information about the disease situation in their territories or cooperate fully with international organizations and other states. Typically, fear of economic damage resulting from the reactions and over-reactions of other states to disease outbreaks motivated states to exercise their sovereignty in non-transparent, uncooperative ways. Countries also tried to hide or downplay infectious disease outbreaks because of concerns about outbreaks tarnishing the images and reputations of the affected nations.

The IHR's collapse as an international legal regime attests to the frequency of state attempts to avoid economic and political fallout from infectious disease epidemics in their territories. The IHR were a Westphalian governance tool because states negotiated and accepted the IHR's disciplines on the exercise of sovereignty with respect to the diseases subject to the Regulations. Frequent violations of the obligations to notify WHO of certain disease outbreaks and to restrict measures in trade and travel to specified actions meant that the disciplines were not effective constraints on the exercise of sovereignty. Sovereignty, even within the framework of Westphalian public health, remained essentially unregulated.

The first two stages of China's response to SARS mirror the historical pattern of the way states exercised their sovereignty in connection with infectious disease problems. China's attempts to hide the outbreak, deny its full scope, provide partial and non-transparent information, and limit cooperation with WHO are all familiar from the history of state responses to epidemics within their borders. Most experts attribute these features of the Chinese response to SARS to China's fears about how full disclosure of the outbreak would affect its economy and growing reputation as a place to invest, do business, and export. Full disclosure about the outbreak would also raise questions about the government's and the Communist Party's policies on public health that neither the government nor the Party wanted to answer.

The pattern of behavior exhibited by China on SARS and by other states during previous outbreaks serves as powerful evidence of the failure of international health governance on infectious diseases developed from 1851. The Westphalian approach to infectious disease control proved inadequate in implementing disciplines that would facilitate effective international action. The failure of Westphalian disciplines points to an underlying problem with the incentives and disincentives states faced when confronted with decisions on how to exercise their sovereignty with respect to epidemics.

The historical pedigree of the pattern of behavior described above means that, over time, states have exercised their sovereignty in a way that inhibits international cooperation and coordination. Under Westphalian public health, the incentives to cooperate apparently did not often outweigh the incentives to minimize damage to a country's reputation and economy by being less than forthright about infectious disease problems. The disincentives for dissimulation, such as the risk of getting caught being less than truthful and uncooperative at the expense of other states, also apparently were not significant enough to alter the rational calculations of states. Such low disincentives connect to the obscure and neglected status of public health as an issue in international relations. The short-term gains from dissimulating on infectious disease outbreaks outweighed any longer-term costs from being seen as selfish in connection with public health issues.

What happened to China in the SARS outbreak deviates from the traditional pattern of Westphalian sovereignty undermining international cooperation. Despite exercising its sovereignty in a manner consistent with applicable international law, the political dynamics of Westphalian public health, and the historical pattern of state behavior during outbreaks, China eventually engaged in an embarrassing and highly damaging retreat. China's retreat cannot be explained by the functioning of international health governance pursuant to the Westphalian model.

Rather, China's retreat occurred because Chinese sovereignty could not withstand the forces brought to bear on China by global health governance.

As explained in Chapter 4, global health governance is a concept that challenges and moves beyond the state-centric approach of Westphalian public health. Global health governance represents a strategy that seeks to build stronger governance roles for non-state actors in international relations. Much of the energy for the movement toward global health governance comes from the realization that state-centric governance approaches, such as the IHR, are inadequate because the state-centric strategy cannot effectively regulate sovereignty. Expecting sovereign states to formulate, accept, and actually obey formal rules of behavior on infectious diseases had, by the 1990s, begun to look like a fool's errand.

As discussed in Chapter 4, prior to the SARS outbreak, WHO had begun to move beyond the state centrism of Westphalian public health with its proposal to include epidemiological information from non-governmental sources in global surveillance efforts. The World Health Assembly approved this policy shift in 2001, and WHO was developing and refining its ability to mine non-governmental sources of information through its Global Outbreak Alert and Response Network (Global Network) before SARS emerged.

China's refusal to provide SARS outbreak information to WHO in a timely, transparent, complete, and verifiable manner ran headlong into the global health governance mechanism of formal integration of non-governmental information into global infectious disease surveillance. Information provided by non-state actors provided the catalyst for WHO and other countries to intensify pressure on the Chinese government, forcing it to retreat repeatedly until the charade could no longer be sustained in any form.

For example, WHO's initial approach to China on 10 February 2003 was provoked not by information coming from the Chinese government but from information provided by non-state actors concerning an outbreak of severe respiratory illness in Guangdong Province. It is not by accident that WHO first approached the Chinese government on the same day (10 February) the WHO office in Beijing received an e-mail from the son of a former WHO employee in China about a worrying outbreak in Guangdong Province (Piller, 2003) and ProMED-mail posted an e-mail asking for information about an epidemic in Guangdong Province being linked in Internet chat rooms to hospital closings and fatalities (ProMED-mail, 2003). Government prohibitions on the media reporting WHO's 15 March global alert did not prevent news of the alert circulating in China by mobile phone, e-mail, and the Internet (Huang, 2003, p. 69). With news of the outbreak in Guangdong Province escaping government attempts to suppress it, China had to respond, in some fashion, to WHO inquiries.

This pattern repeated itself a number of times during China's response to SARS. The accusations of a prominent Chinese physician and Communist Party member on 9 April that the Chinese government was not telling the truth about the number of SARS cases in Beijing provided momentum for WHO's insistence that the Chinese government permit it to investigate the Beijing outbreak. The physician's accusations 'were posted on the Internet and became the talk of Beijing' (Pomfret, 2003p). Unofficial information provided by Chinese physicians also undermined the government's claims about the number of SARS cases in Beijing, helping create the context in which WHO issued its highly unusual public criticism of the Chinese government on 16 April. The flow of non-governmental information materially advanced the progress of WHO's investigations on the SARS outbreak in China. In the battle to control information about SARS, China was always on the defensive.

This analysis does not mean that WHO depended only on non-state actors to provide information about SARS during the global campaign to control the epidemic. Other countries significantly affected by SARS openly shared information on SARS cases with WHO and cooperated closely with WHO in containing SARS. The global campaign against SARS benefited greatly from such government-provided epidemiological information. WHO personnel in Asia also contributed to the surveillance and response effort, as Dr Carlo Urbani's work in Vietnam illustrated. Global surveillance for SARS comprised a mosaic of different sources of information that was valuable to the global effort to contain the spread of SARS.

With China, however, the non-governmental sources of information proved critical in the face of Chinese official intransigence to come clean on the extent of the SARS problem. Unlike past situations of governmental denial and difficult behavior in outbreak situations, on this occasion WHO had stronger epidemiological and political positions vis-à-vis China.

Epidemiologically, WHO's ability to gather and use information from non-governmental sources helped the Organization develop arguments about the outbreak in China that proved extremely powerful in WHO's dealings with the Chinese government. Politically, the World Health Assembly's 2001 approval of WHO collection and use of non-governmental sources of information strengthened WHO in its use of such information with respect to China's SARS outbreak. The SARS outbreak illustrates the power of the global health governance strategy of bringing non-state actors into the process of global infectious disease surveillance.

The premise behind expanding global surveillance to include non-governmental sources of information was that countries can no longer hide outbreaks from the world because of the revolution in information technologies. As a WHO consultation on the revision of the IHR stated in 1995, 'in this age of wide media coverage, nothing can be hidden' (WHO, 1995, p. 10). The globalization of information facilitated by new information technologies, such as the Internet and e-mail, radically transformed the political context in which states exercised their public health sovereignty. Incentives to cover up or deny outbreaks disappear when cover-up and denial are doomed to rapid, embarrassing, and damaging failure.

Expanding infectious disease surveillance from reliance only on governmental information to include non-governmental sources of epidemiological data merely reflects the reality of an increasingly globalized world. As WHO (2003b, p. 8) stated in May 2003 reflections on lessons learned from SARS:

> This is the most important lesson for all nations: in a globalized, electronically connected world, attempts to conceal cases of an infectious disease, for fear of economic and social consequences, must be recognized as a short-term stop-gap measure that carries a very high price – loss of credibility in the eyes of the international community, escalating negative domestic economic impact, damage to health and economics of neighboring countries, and a very real risk that outbreaks within the country's own territory can spiral out of control.

Most of the international community recognized this lesson when the World Health Assembly approved WHO's use of non-governmental information for surveillance purposes in 2001, and virtually all SARS-affected countries acted in accordance with this lesson in their handling of SARS. Technological transformations altered the environment in which states faced the sovereign decision whether to be open or closed concerning infectious disease outbreaks. Under the Westphalian model, this sovereign decision was only constrained by rules of international law, which were of limited application and of even more limited utility. Bringing non-governmental sources of information to bear on surveillance has forced sovereignty to transition into a much more demanding and unforgiving environment.

The SARS outbreak witnessed the humbling of China's sovereignty by global health governance. In the Westphalian framework, sovereignty is supreme power over territory; and such supreme power extends to the generation and dissemination of information. Efforts by China to maintain control over SARS information within its territory failed badly. As the *Washington Post* reported, the Chinese 'government could not control the dissemination of information to the World Health Organization' (Pomfret, 2003p). The loss of control of epidemiological information in the SARS outbreak represents an excellent case study of one of the defining characteristics of globalization – the sovereign state increasingly loses control over politics, economics, and culture within its own territory. Issues and problems become denationalized or deterritorialized, which renders the traditional exercise of Westphalian sovereignty ineffective, counter-productive, and harmful to others. China's behavior in the SARS outbreak provides further evidence that globalization alters the context in which states exercise their sovereignty and perhaps alters the very concept of sovereignty itself.

Ironically, the SARS outbreak represented China's second major mishandling of infectious disease surveillance and response in recent years. In 2001, China admitted that the HIV/AIDS problem in its territory was far worse than it previously acknowledged. A UNAIDS assessment of the HIV/AIDS epidemic in China conducted at the end of 2001 argued that China was 'on the verge of a catastrophe that could result in unimaginable human suffering, economic loss and social devastation' and was 'witnessing the unfolding of an HIV/AIDS epidemic of proportions beyond belief, an epidemic that calls for an urgent and proper, but currently yet unanswered quintessential response' (UNAIDS, 2002c, p. 7). The same UNAIDS study observed that, in China, '[c]ensorship and restrictions on information concerning HIV/AIDS severely hinders an effective response' (UNAIDS, 2002c, p. 70).

Yet, in spite of the embarrassing revelation about the extent of the HIV/AIDS problem in China and UNAIDS' criticism of China's censorship of HIV/AIDS-related information, in 2002 China detained a prominent HIV/AIDS activist, Wan Yanhai, for distributing by e-mail government information on the true scale of the HIV/AIDS epidemic in Henan Province, the epicenter of HIV transmission through unsanitary blood transfusions at government-run clinics (Pan, 2002). In an editorial, the *Washington Post* observed that a 'striking conclusion that emerges from Dr. Wan's disappearance, aside from the atmosphere of secrecy, is how shortsighted are the regime's policies. Facing the risk of an Africa-style AIDS crisis that could decimate its population and economy, any forward-looking government would welcome the efforts of such activists' (*Washington Post,* 2002).

As was the case with SARS, China was under no international legal obligation to report HIV/AIDS cases to WHO or UNAIDS, or to engage in international cooperation on the Chinese HIV/AIDS problem. Resonance with the Westphalian framework did not, however, spare China from being subjected to intense and withering scrutiny of its governance approach to HIV/AIDS because the international community had information about the growing scale of the Chinese HIV/AIDS epidemic. This incident also reveals the futility of Westphalian concepts of public health sovereignty in a world of globalized information on infectious diseases.

China's mishandling of SARS demonstrated that it still had not grasped the new context for public health governance – epidemiological information about germs does not recognize borders. In connection to SARS, China played the sovereignty card only to retreat when its sovereignty was seen, again, to be a deliberate attempt to hide an outbreak about which the world already knew. In some respects, China's behavior with respect to SARS was more inexplicable than with HIV/AIDS because SARS-CoV, unlike HIV, is more transmissible through respiratory means and thus was dangerous in a world dependent on global air travel.

Both on its own and in combination with HIV/AIDS, the Chinese approach to SARS raised questions about why China exercised its sovereignty on public health issues in the ways it did. Much commentary on the Chinese response to SARS focused on the nature of Communist Party rule and how such rule played a major role in China's historic miscalculations on SARS. In the Westphalian template, the nature of a state's government or ideology is not an issue because the principles of sovereignty and non-intervention mean that a state is free to determine its own political and economic structures. Whether a government is a democracy by the people or a dictatorship of the proletariat does not matter in Westphalian public health. Post-Westphalian public health does not share this agnosticism. Global health governance contains assumptions about what constitutes 'good governance' and how such governance is achieved.

For example, in its report on the HIV/AIDS crisis in China, UNAIDS (2002c, p. 70) argued that 'good governance and sustainable human development are indivisible and represent each other's underpinnings.... Therefore a successful response to HIV/AIDS is strongly linked to sustainable human development and good governance.' UNAIDS (2002c, p. 70) described good governance with respect to HIV/AIDS as follows:

'Worldwide, societal openness, transparency and broad participation of people living with or affected by HIV/AIDS have shown over and over to be at the core of effective HIV/AIDS responses.' Similarly, Human Rights Watch (2003, p. 28) observed: 'International experience with the HIV/AIDS pandemic over the past two decades has shown that the ability to share and access information (central to freedom of expression) has been absolutely essential for rights and improvements in treatment for those with the virus or disease as well as to any successful prevention program.' For China, 'important aspects of good governance in relation to the response to HIV/AIDS are the access to free flow of information, greater involvement of civil society and affected people in the processes of decision making regarding HIV/AIDS prevention and care' (UNAIDS, 2002c, p. 70). This concept of 'good governance' does not stop at the border but pierces sovereignty in order to focus on internal methods of addressing infectious disease problems.

The concept of global health governance maintains that increasing the quantity and quality of global surveillance requires openness, transparency, and wide participation in public health within and among countries in the collection, analysis, and dissemination of epidemiological information. The involvement of non-governmental actors in global health governance mechanisms alters the Westphalian linkage of sovereignty with formal governments and makes sovereignty more participatory and accountable. Global health governance requires political recognition of, and commitment to, an 'open public health society' in which (1) citizens have a right to receive and disseminate information important to the protection and promotion of their health; and (2) non-state actors can hold governments accountable for their management of the public's health. In short, global health governance requires the exercise of a *certain kind of sovereignty*, which differs radically from the Westphalian approach to sovereignty.

The Chinese handling of both its HIV/AIDS and SARS epidemics reflects, however, an antithetical governance philosophy to the one promulgated by the notion of global health governance. Under Chinese law and Communist Party policy, information about infectious disease epidemics is considered a state secret (Huang, 2003; Mirsky, 2003; Pomfret, 2003r); and people, such as Wan Yanhai, who reveal state secrets can be subject to arrest and punishment. Laurie Garrett (2003) reported that her Chinese journalist contacts indicated that the reporters in Guangdong Province who published stories on the outbreak in February 2003 were 'severely repressed' for these actions. Human Rights Watch (2003, p. 28) argued that, in China, the rights to freedom of expression, association, and assembly are routinely violated in connection with HIV/AIDS. The Chinese approach to epidemics is, thus, light years from the template for 'good governance' prescribed by the concept of global health governance.

These deeper political implications of global health governance help explain why China's mishandling of the SARS outbreak provided commentators with material for critically analyzing China's communist rule. The SARS outbreak made the Communist Party and its leadership appear woefully out of touch with the globalized context of public health. The *Washington Post* reported that 'China's response to SARS has angered and befuddled Western scientists and policymakers' (Pomfret, 2003h). The *Wall Street Journal* observed that '[t]he Chinese response to SARS looks like a textbook case of how not to react to a public health emergency' (Fritsch, Pottinger, and Chang, 2003).

In critical discourse on China's response to SARS, the culprit was not a novel, respiratory pathogen against which public health officials had no diagnostic, therapeutic, or vaccine responses; the culprit of the mess in China was communism. As the *Washington Post* stated, '[f]rom the start, China's reaction to the disease was textbook Chinese communism' (Pomfret, 2003h). Xu Wenli, one of the founders of the democracy movement in China, noted that 'while SARS is a frightening phenomenon, a political system in such a condition that it would hide a dangerous disease from its own people and from the world is far more frightening' (Xu, 2003). Commenting on the SARS outbreak, an editorial in the *Wall Street Journal* argues that 'China's other disease is its secretive dictatorship' (*Wall Street Journal*, 2003b). Echoing the tenets of 'good governance' for public health, Anthony Saich (2003) argued that 'China's new leaders need to draw the lesson that for continued rapid economic growth they must allow greater freedom of information, reduce coercion, promote transparency and enhance accountability.' The verdict rendered by many commentators was that communism proved itself ill-equipped to manage sovereignty in the context of globalized anarchy.

Literature critical of China's response to SARS frequently raised the question of whether the SARS outbreak would represent 'China's Chernobyl' (*The Economist*, 2003, p. 9; *Washington Post*, 2003b; Goldgeier, 2003). Making the analogy between the Chernobyl disaster in the Soviet Union in 1986 and the SARS outbreak in China focused attention on whether SARS would trigger a cascade of reforms that could weaken communist control and introduce and nurture forms of more democratic governance. *The Economist* (2003, p. 9) succinctly captured the analogy:

> The [Chernobyl] explosion...is now regarded as a great accelerator of the programmes of *glasnost* and *perestroika*, of 'openness' and 're-structuring.' These helped, just three years later, to bring down first the Soviet empire, then the Soviet Union itself and the Communist Party. So is SARS China's Chernobyl; or will the chain-reaction this time be controlled?

For purposes of my analysis, whether SARS will eventually have the impact on communist rule in China that many believe Chernobyl had on communism in the Soviet Union is not the central issue. The analogy, at present, is interesting speculation; but not enough time has passed to move much beyond speculation. Cogent arguments have been made that SARS will not represent China's Chernobyl. Saich (2003) argued, for example, that '[a]s China's leaders begin to win their war against severe acute respiratory syndrome (Sars), the prospect of a dramatic systemic change – the "Chernobyl factor" – looks remote' because '"old politics" has...reasserted itself,...while the party as a whole is extolling its virtues in taming the viral beast.' Evidence is already appearing that China may return to heavy-handed censorship to prevent public debate and discussion about political reform, shutting the window of opportunity for less restricted speech created by the SARS crisis (Pomfret, 2003t).

In addition, the impact of Chernobyl on Soviet communism might be more symbolic than substantive. The Chernobyl disaster was a symbol of a sick and dying political system. Chernobyl was not the source of the sickness and terminal illness, only a particularly memorable symptom. Chernobyl occurred as the Soviet Union accelerated toward its ultimate demise, a horrific accident revealing why this great power was headed for the ash heap of history. By contrast, SARS hit China as a rising great power in international relations. At the end of the day, the Chernobyl analogy does not take critical analysis very far.

What is more relevant for my analysis is the mere fact that the Chernobyl–SARS analogy was made so frequently. The analogy itself supports the argument that public health has moved beyond the Westphalian framework. The criticisms heaped on the Communist Party in China because of its response to SARS illustrate the more demanding procedural and substantive nature of global health governance. In Westphalian public health, sovereignty presumes supreme power over information within the state's territory; and how a state regulated the flow of information within its territory was not an issue of diplomatic concern. Global health governance on infectious diseases sweeps this

Westphalian presumption aside and demands openness, transparency, accountability, and international cooperation on surveillance and response. Any country that tightly controls information about infectious diseases within its territory would find this sovereign choice significantly challenged by the surveillance dynamic created by global health governance. China's loss of control over epidemic information on both HIV/AIDS and SARS shows how radically the post-Westphalian context of public health challenged, penetrated, and exploded Chinese public health sovereignty.

As the Chernobyl–SARS analogy indicates, exploding public health sovereignty reverberates throughout China's governing system and political ideology. This reverberation may or may not contribute to more general challenges to communist rule in China and systemic liberalization of the political regime, but the fact that a public health emergency triggered wide-ranging criticism of a rising great power's governance and ideological system further demonstrates the emergence of post-Westphalian public health. In the Westphalian system of international politics, public health was not on the agenda of 'high politics' and represented an obscure, neglected area of international relations. In addition, infectious disease problems did not produce a political dynamic through which the sovereignty of great powers could be challenged. For China, the SARS outbreak became a matter of 'high politics' and a crisis for this rising great power's government, leadership, ideology, and sovereignty. As Huang Yanzhong (2003, p. 71) argued, '[t]he SARS epidemic is not simply a public health problem; it has caused the most severe socio-political crisis for the Chinese leadership since the 1989 Tianamen Square crackdown.'

As Chapter 8 explores in more detail, my argument that global health governance trumped Chinese sovereignty during the SARS outbreak is not an argument about the 'end of sovereignty' in global public health. The main point about this trumping is that the conception of sovereignty embedded in Westphalian public health has been superseded, through global health governance, by an epidemiological and political context that demands that sovereignty be exercised in certain ways. These demands represent disciplines on the exercise of sovereignty that do not emanate from formal international legal agreements, which were the main source of disciplines on Westphalian sovereignty. The disciplines flow from the growth of globalized interactions among states and peoples, transformations in information technologies, and deliberate policy choices to expand surveillance to include non-governmental sources of information.

A final feature of global health governance's trumping of Chinese sovereignty involves the changed role of WHO in the post-Westphalian context of public health. A striking element of the SARS saga in China is the power exercised by WHO. As indicated earlier, international organizations traditionally have not publicly confronted and embarrassed member states during controversies, and particularly not member states that are great powers. This Westphalian approach of international organizations toward their member states did not characterize what happened between WHO and China during the SARS outbreak. Chapter 5's narrative of the SARS epidemic reveals WHO's growing confrontational attitude toward China, leading to WHO's publicly delivered rebuke on 16 April 2003.

This rebuke is dramatic in its own right, but behind the rebuke are deeper developments that connect to global health governance. The highly fragmented nature of political authority in the Westphalian framework concentrates authority for public health inside sovereign states, with international health organizations only possessing very limited authority defined by formal treaties. Literature on the globalization of public health points out that public health risks and resources increasingly escape the ability of sovereign states to control on their own. The typical policy response reached in analysis of the globalization of public health is advocacy for broader, deeper, and better international cooperation among states.

Informing arguments for improved international cooperation was a sense, not always made explicit, that tinkering with the traditional Westphalian framework would not be sufficient for addressing globalized public health risks. As Chapter 4 explored, the concept of global health governance emerged as a strategy to move public health beyond the state-centric system. Although much attention focused, quite rightly, on the involvement of non-state actors, global health governance as a concept had significant implications for WHO as the leading international health organization. Building non-state actors more directly into public health governance requires organization and coordination functions that no single sovereign state could shoulder. Tapping non-governmental sources of epidemiological information also requires authoritative vetting of such information to ensure that accurate, verifiable data is separated from unsupported rumors.

In many respects, the heightened importance of WHO in coordinating global surveillance mirrors the functional need states realized in the late nineteenth and early twentieth centuries that international cooperation on infectious diseases required a permanent, central international organization. At both the 1874 and 1881 international sanitary conferences, delegates discussed the creation of a permanent international health organization to facilitate cooperation on infectious diseases (Fidler, 1999, pp. 47–8). Although nothing came of these efforts, the creation of four international health organizations in the first 25 years of the twentieth century attests to the importance states placed on the existence of international organizations to assist states to cooperate on infectious disease control.

The same functional need for WHO exists in today's world of globalized anarchy. Given the expansion of surveillance to include non-governmental sources, the need for WHO leadership and capabilities in this area is increased. Casting the surveillance net wider gives WHO better information and opportunities to work with states to intervene more rapidly and effectively against outbreaks. In addition, WHO (2002d, p. 7) stresses that a key feature of its activities under the Global Network is to protect states from the potential harmful impact of unverified news stories or rumors of outbreaks circulating in global communication networks.

Before SARS, WHO was beginning to shoulder the organizational, coordination, and verification functions produced by the global health governance strategy. The SARS outbreak highlighted the increased responsibility and power WHO has in post-Westphalian infectious disease control. (See also Chapter 7's discussion of WHO's issuance of travel advisories as evidence of the Organization's increased importance and power in post-Westphalian public health governance.) WHO's handling of China's recalcitrance also serves as evidence of how global health governance increases the importance and power of WHO compared with WHO's constrained role and reality in the Westphalian framework.

National interest v. global public goods for health

China's confrontation with public health's 'new world order' involves another feature of post-Westphalian public health that China failed to grasp – the importance of global public goods for health (GPGH). The first two stages of China's response to SARS revealed its leaders pursuing a narrowly constructed national interest. Until the policy collapsed under the weight of its own deceit, China approached SARS in a hyper-introverted manner, almost as if the rest of the world did not exist or have legitimate concerns about China's behavior. The first two stages of China's response exhibited the Chinese government's myopic focus on 'social stability' in China, continued trade and investment flows into China, and the power and image of the Communist Party.

Even in the face of a novel, respiratory pathogen spreading rapidly and China's increasing integration with the globalizing world, China behaved as if its national interest could be constructed and pursued without serious consideration of the concerns of other countries and non-state actors, such as multinational corporations (MNCs) and non-governmental organizations (NGOs). China's conception of its national interest shattered in the post-Westphalian atmosphere of SARS.

Westphalian public health permitted states to construct national interests narrowly because the formal disciplines on the exercise of sovereignty required little from states. These disciplines focused on how infectious disease outbreaks might affect the mechanistic interactions of states, leaving considerable room for countries to construct their national interests on public health without the need to consider significantly the concerns of other nations. Westphalian principles, such as non-intervention, bolstered the ability states had to craft their national interests on infectious diseases narrowly.

China's narrow construction of its national interest in the SARS outbreak ran headlong into the much less forgiving, more demanding context of post-Westphalian public health. The shift to global health governance in infectious disease surveillance and response changed the ground rules for sovereign states. Expanding global surveillance to include non-governmental sources of information seeks to improve the quantity and quality of infectious disease surveillance. As Giesecke (2003, p. 209) argued, 'open reporting and sharing of information on outbreaks, which makes it possible for the international community to eliminate them early[,] is a clear GPGH.'

The SARS outbreak demonstrates the same thing – improved global surveillance represents a GPGH that benefits governments, MNCs, NGOs, and individuals. China's decision not to contribute to the production of timely and accurate global surveillance on SARS undermined this GPGH and alienated the Chinese government from the global community. China's short-sighted approach to its national interest backfired badly because it proved incapable, during the first two stages of its response, of understanding its role in, and responsibility for, the production of a GPGH.

Just as global health governance proved more demanding of sovereignty than Westphalian public health, the GPGH concept reflects a radically different context in which states formulate their national interests with respect to infectious diseases. As the collapse in tourist trade to China and fears of SARS in the foreign business community demonstrated, China's crafting of its national interest could not be state-centric in orientation. Chinese participation in the GPGH of global surveillance was perhaps as important in reassuring non-state actors as it was for Chinese relations with fellow sovereign states. This reality again reflects the post-Westphalian environment of global public health.

As with the confrontation between Chinese sovereignty and global health governance, the collapse of China's initial framing of its national interest in SARS has deeper political implications. The idea that a country's national interest with respect to infectious diseases can no longer be narrowly tailored and insular is not new. Many states affected by SARS took a globalized approach to their national interests and, thus, contributed proactively to the GPGH of global SARS surveillance.

One aspect of Singapore's behavior provides an excellent example of a country formulating its national interest in harmony with the globalized reality of the SARS threat. WHO initially scheduled Singapore's removal from the list of SARS-affected countries on 11 May. Such removal would have represented WHO's clean bill of health for Singapore and a testament to Singapore's efforts to contain SARS. Shortly before removal from the list of SARS-affected areas, Singapore identified one new case. Disclosure of the case would delay Singapore's removal from the list of SARS-affected areas, and such delay could prove economically expensive as tourists and business might continue to stay away. Despite temptations not to disclose this new case, Singapore reported the case to WHO. WHO did not remove Singapore from the list of SARS-affected areas until 31 May because of this one case. This incident illustrates Singapore's formulation of its national interest in a manner that fully reflected the importance of the GPGH of accurate global SARS surveillance.

Singapore's commitment to global SARS surveillance stands in stark contrast to China's repeated, calculated, and futile efforts to deny and cover up the SARS problem within its borders. While Singapore responded impressively to the post-Westphalian climate of infectious disease control, China's construction of its national interest in the same climate was surreal. Of the countries and areas hit hard by SARS, China alone adopted an attitude completely out of touch with epidemiological and political realities. The fact that all other SARS-affected countries participated actively in the production of the GPGH of global SARS surveillance is impressive evidence of post-Westphalian public health. Countries produced this GPGH despite the complete absence of any rules of international law applicable to the crisis. The formulation of national interests in many countries harmonized rapidly around the WHO strategy for global SARS control. Such harmonization of national public health policy in the face of an infectious disease threat is truly remarkable.

China's conspicuous place outside the harmonization of national interests that occurred raises more questions about communism's ability to understand post-Westphalian public health governance. The diversity of government types among the countries that developed harmonized national interests suggests that China's failure cannot be attributed to authoritarianism alone. China's Communist Party proved painfully incapable of crafting the country's national interest in a manner that reflected the globalized reality of China's place in the world. China's success at containing SARS after its policy reversal does not redeem the Communist Party's monumental miscalculation.

These observations connect with the arguments about SARS as 'China's Chernobyl' described earlier. Running through both sets of arguments is the common concern with Chinese communism's inability to adjust to the demands of post-Westphalian public health. For historical and ideological reasons, China has long exhibited sensitivity about outside interests interfering with its sovereignty. China has also prided itself on forging political and economic systems that exhibit 'Chinese characteristics.' These Chinese tendencies fit the Westphalian framework well but appear as anachronistic and illegitimate phobias in the context of post-Westphalian public health. Communist China has yet to demonstrate that it grasps how embedded the Middle Kingdom is in global public health. The SARS outbreak teaches the lesson that the formulation of the national interest about germs cannot recognize physical and ideological borders.

SARS, China, and Taiwan

China's confrontation with public health's 'new world order' also involves the impact of SARS on China's traditional notions of sovereignty and national interest with respect to Taiwan. China fiercely defends its claim to sovereignty over Taiwan, leading some experts to worry that China will risk war to preserve sovereignty over Taiwan. China's uncompromising approach to Taiwan has also involved China opposing and blocking any formal or informal connections between Taiwan and any entity within the United Nations' system. For this reason, Taiwan has had no contact or relationship with WHO since Taiwan lost its United Nations membership to China three decades ago.

China's unbending position on Taiwan created problems for Taiwan's handling of its SARS outbreak. As Chapter 5 described, Taiwan's SARS epidemic grew worse in May 2003, leading to Taiwan requiring more international assistance. International help for Taiwan early in its outbreak came bilaterally from the United States because China blocked WHO assistance. The deterioration of the SARS situation in Taiwan in May 2003 confronted China's Taiwan policy with a dilemma. In May 2003, the SARS outbreak bent the unbendable as China permitted a WHO team to travel to Taiwan to provide outbreak assistance. As noted in *The Lancet*, the WHO team's visit to Taiwan 'was a historic moment: the first visit by any representative of a UN-affiliated organization since China took Taiwan's seat on the world body 30 years ago' (Watts, 2003, p. 1709).

This development illustrates the power of post-Westphalian public health to challenge states in deeply and fiercely held political positions. The SARS outbreak did not break the political deadlock over Taiwan between Beijing and Taipei. Because of Chinese opposition, WHO rebuffed Taiwan's attempts to use the SARS crisis to gain formal observer status at WHO. But China's refusal to allow WHO to interact with Taiwan could not withstand the political pressure SARS placed on China. Chinese leaders probably realized that continuing to prohibit WHO assistance for Taiwan would only exacerbate the terrible situation China had produced in its reaction to SARS. Even China's uncompromising stance on Taiwan could not stand in the way of the need to incorporate Taiwan into the global effort to bring SARS under control.

Conclusion

As the epidemiological and governance epicenter of the SARS outbreak, China played a critical role in the global effort against SARS. China's behavior jeopardized this effort until the country retreated in the face of the consequences of its terrible miscalculations. This retreat tells the story of the humbling of the sovereignty and ideology of one of the world's rising great powers. For this reason alone, the episode is unprecedented in the history of international efforts on infectious disease control.

China's response to SARS makes public health history in other ways as well. The emergence of SARS as a threat would have severely challenged public health governance regardless of China's behavior. The nature of China's response dramatically increased the governance stakes of the SARS outbreak, which makes the global campaign's triumph over SARS all the more stunning.

Equally important and historic is the fact that global health governance and GPGH routed China's exercise of sovereignty and formulation of narrow, insular national interests. Nothing in this confrontation followed the tenets and patterns of Westphalian public health. As much or more than anything else, China's capitulation to the dynamics of public health's 'new world order' confirms SARS as the first post-Westphalian pathogen and the coming-of-age of a governance strategy for infectious diseases more radical than any previous governance innovation in this area of international relations.

7

Beyond China: Lessons from SARS for Post-Westphalian Public Health

Introduction

Although China provides the most dramatic evidence that public health has moved into a post-Westphalian context, the SARS outbreak produced other indications that public health has transitioned into a new governance era. These developments demonstrate that SARS has governance implications that reach beyond China's handling of SARS. The manner in which SARS was managed globally reveals the emergence of a framework of universal scope affecting all countries, be they weak or powerful. This chapter analyzes four features of the SARS outbreak that support the argument that public health governance has entered a post-Westphalian period.

Strengthening global health governance on infectious diseases

Chapter 4 argued that global health governance was one of the main concepts developing in the 1990s and early 2000s in response to the threats posed by emerging and re-emerging infectious diseases. Chapter 6 demonstrated that global health governance trumped the Westphalian exercise of Chinese sovereignty during the SARS outbreak. The SARS outbreak witnessed the strengthening of global health governance in broader ways that connect with the pre-SARS development of this concept and the clash between Chinese sovereignty and global health governance.

In the context of infectious disease control, a key feature of global health governance that emerged in the 1990s was the direct involvement of non-state actors in surveillance for outbreaks and disease events.

As explained in Chapter 4, in its revision of the International Health Regulations (IHR), WHO sought to strengthen this regime by allowing WHO to collect, analyze, and use epidemiological information supplied by non-governmental sources. WHO moved more aggressively in this direction by establishing its Global Outbreak Alert and Response Network (Global Network) in 1997, well before the revised IHR were finished. World Health Assembly approval of this shift in surveillance came in 2001. The SARS outbreak vindicated WHO's move to include non-governmental sources of information in global surveillance.

This vindication comes from what happened with respect to not only China (analyzed in Chapter 6) but also other countries affected by SARS. Reporting of SARS cases to WHO by affected countries did not follow the pattern that unfortunately developed under the IHR. As explored in Chapter 3, WHO member states routinely failed to notify WHO of outbreaks of diseases subject to the IHR. The general and consistent pattern of state behavior in the Westphalian system was not to report disease events to WHO and other countries. Exactly the opposite occurred in the SARS outbreak.

In light of the history of the failure of disease reporting obligations under international law, what happened in the SARS outbreak is remarkable. Despite being under no international legal obligation to report SARS cases to WHO, virtually all countries afflicted by SARS notified WHO of cases rapidly, continuously, and transparently. Public health experts have praised countries as diverse as Canada, Singapore, and Vietnam for their reporting of SARS cases.

The example of Singapore's reporting of a new case on the very day it was scheduled to be taken off WHO's list of SARS-affected areas described in Chapter 6 serves as a powerful illustration of a new attitude toward global disease notifications than that which prevailed in the era of Westphalian public health. Many countries that faced the same decision as China on SARS reporting opted for openness, transparency, and cooperation without being under any international legal obligation to act in this manner.

The pattern of open disease reporting experienced in the SARS outbreak tells a tale of improved *government* participation in global epidemiological surveillance. How, then, does improved government behavior represent evidence of the strengthening of global health governance, with its emphasis on the involvement of non-state actors? This question prompts two replies.

First, global health governance does not exclude improvements in public health governance within governments and between governments.

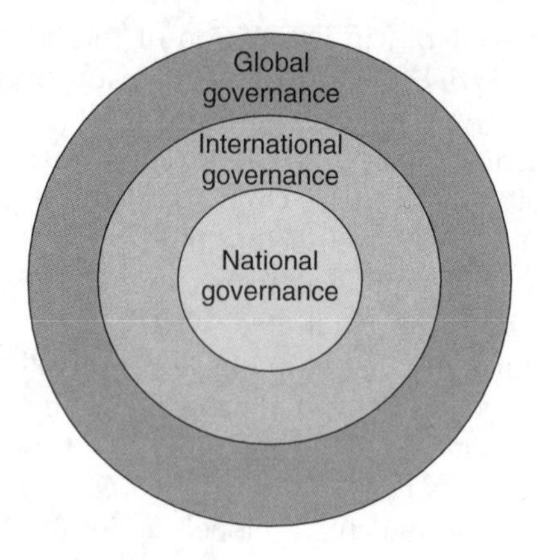

Figure 7.1 Public health governance

Better national governance and international governance on infectious disease control contributes positively to global health governance. Governance for public health resembles a series of concentric circles (see Figure 7.1). The governmental break from the Westphalian pattern of non-reporting does not diminish the importance of global health governance in the SARS outbreak.

Second, the improved pattern of government participation seen with SARS is directly related to WHO's ability to gather non-governmental information about outbreaks. The move to include non-governmental sources of information as part of epidemiological surveillance had two fundamental motivations: (1) to harness the potential of new information technologies for public health; and (2) to overcome the historical pattern of sovereign states not reporting infectious disease outbreaks, even when international law required them to do so. The overall strategy aimed to transform the incentives sovereign states had in connection with the decision to report disease events. The Westphalian pattern of non-reporting reflected incentives driving states not to be transparent and open with respect to epidemiological information. The post-Westphalian involvement of non-state actors in disease surveillance would, the hope was, reverse the incentives such that states would report rather than hide outbreaks.

The sustained level of open reporting of SARS cases by virtually all SARS-affected countries provides powerful evidence that global health governance has indeed shifted the incentives. Except for China, all other SARS-affected countries decided to exercise their sovereignty by reporting SARS cases to WHO. Sovereign calculations of the national interest produced a pattern of open reporting to which developed and developing, liberal and authoritarian, states contributed. Informing these calculations was the realization that hiding SARS cases would be futile and counter-productive in an age in which non-state actors can globally disseminate disease information. Confirmation of this realization was at hand in the disastrous and humiliating efforts of China to cover up the scale of its SARS problem.

WHO's work prior to SARS to incorporate non-governmental sources of information into global surveillance may have begun the process of convincing states that hiding outbreaks was no longer possible or preferable. WHO had, thus, laid the groundwork for states to break with the Westphalian pattern of non-reporting. At the May 2003 World Health Assembly meeting, WHO member states reaffirmed the importance of WHO's ability to use information from non-governmental sources. The World Health Assembly requested the WHO Director-General 'to take into account reports from sources other than official notification' (World Health Assembly, 2003b). This request marked the second time the World Health Assembly has supported expanding global infectious disease surveillance to include non-governmental sources of information; but, coming in the midst of the SARS crisis, the May 2003 action by the World Health Assembly carries much more political significance. The World Health Assembly significantly strengthened the global health governance strategy WHO pioneered with its Global Network.

China's behavior during the SARS outbreak elucidates why the World Health Assembly's action is politically important for future global health governance on infectious diseases. China's recalcitrance and deception brought home the importance for global public health of WHO having access to non-governmental sources of information. As noted above, the pre-SARS move toward including non-state actors in global infectious disease surveillance sought to provide WHO and other states with more leverage in confronting countries that hid or denied outbreaks within their territories.

China's behavior put the final nail in the coffin of basing global surveillance for infectious diseases only on governmental information. Given the cooperation exhibited by virtually all other countries afflicted by SARS, the World Health Assembly's renewed support for WHO's use of non-governmental sources of epidemiological information indicates how important such information was to overcoming China's intransigence. In light of the humbling of Chinese sovereignty, the World Health

Assembly's action stands as a warning to any government tempted to behave when a future outbreak occurs as China did on SARS.

The World Health Assembly's action also stands for the coming of age of global health governance for infectious disease surveillance. Although WHO was moving in this direction prior to SARS, the SARS outbreak elevated the global health governance strategy at the heart of the Global Network to a dominant place in the critical area of surveillance. The limited international governance embedded in the IHR's rules on disease notification no longer controls this area of public health policy. Sovereign states no longer monopolize information flows related to infectious disease events.

This loss of exclusive control involves both practical and policy components. As a practical matter, the development of new information technologies makes it nearly impossible, as China discovered, for a sovereign state to control epidemiological information within its borders. But perhaps more significant is the policy component. WHO member states have, twice, approved the legitimacy of incorporating non-governmental information into infectious disease surveillance. This policy move cannot be reconciled with the state-centrism of Westphalian public health but confirms the transition of public health into a post-Westphalian period characterized by global health governance on infectious disease surveillance.

The SARS outbreak strengthened global health governance in another important way. As mentioned in Chapter 6, the SARS outbreak witnessed WHO exercising power and authority unprecedented in the history of this international organization. Chapter 6 focused on how WHO confronted China publicly and rebuked it for its deceptive behavior with respect to SARS. The SARS outbreak contains other evidence of WHO's authority growing in ways unimaginable in the Westphalian framework. This evidence involves the various global alerts and travel advisories WHO issued during the SARS outbreak.

WHO's first global alert, on 12 March 2003, was designed to alert national public health authorities of the international spread of an atypical pneumonia so that such authorities could heighten awareness within their own surveillance and response systems (WHO, 2003j). The 15 March emergency travel advisory contained 'emergency travel recommendations to alert health authorities, physicians, and the traveling public to what was now perceived to be a worldwide threat to health' (WHO, 2003k). WHO later issued travel recommendations that travelers postpone non-essential travel to Hong Kong, Guangdong Province, Beijing, Shanxi Province, Toronto, Tianjin, Inner Mongolia, Taipei, Heibei

Province, and Taiwan (WHO, 2003y-2). The global alert, the emergency travel advisory, and the geographically-specific travel recommendations constituted unprecedented actions by WHO and represent further evidence of a transition to post-Westphalian public health.

WHO's ability and authority to issue such alerts, advisories, and recommendations was not a product of the Westphalian public health template because neither the WHO Constitution nor the IHR invested WHO with this power. The World Health Assembly had not adopted any decisions or recommendations in this area. As Health Canada's National Advisory Committee on SARS and Public Health observed, WHO issued travel advisories during SARS 'without explicit authorization by member states' (National Advisory Committee, 2003, p. 199). Under the Westphalian approach, WHO disseminated government-provided information on areas affected by quarantinable diseases to WHO member states, which then decided whether to apply measures or issue recommendations to persons arriving from or traveling to such areas. In other words, the Westphalian approach about whether to act in ways that may adversely affect trade and travel between countries left such decisions in the hands of sovereign states.

During the SARS outbreak, national governments still made recommendations to their citizens not to travel to certain SARS-affected countries. Radical change occurred when WHO issued alerts, advisories, and recommendations without any express permission or authority to do so under international law or pursuant to policy action by the World Health Assembly. These actions by WHO powerfully indicate that the governance context for infectious diseases had changed. WHO's role in Westphalian public health was to act as a conduit for epidemiological information not to take a strong position on how member states should respond to such information.

Examples from the IHR and HIV/AIDS help illustrate the Westphalian context in which WHO operated prior to SARS. The IHR contained rules restricting how WHO member states could respond to trade and travelers coming from countries afflicted by a disease subject to the Regulations. WHO member states routinely violated these rules, and WHO only infrequently made statements about the appropriate public health response.

For example, in 1998, when the European Union banned the importation of fresh fish products from East African countries suffering a cholera outbreak, WHO (1998) publicly stated that trade embargoes were 'not an appropriate course of action to prevent the international spread of cholera, and can represent an additional burden on the economy of the affected countries.' This statement was a recommendation, based on the legal obligations found in the IHR, to WHO member states about the proper way to respond to cholera outbreaks in other countries. In keeping with the historical patterns seen in the IHR, the European Union ignored this recommendation.

With respect to HIV/AIDS, WHO has been active on its own and then in cooperation with UNAIDS in encouraging states to respond to HIV/AIDS in accordance with principles derived from international human rights law, particularly the principle of non-discrimination. Recommendations on HIV/AIDS have not had any basis in the IHR because HIV/AIDS is not a disease subject to the Regulations, but WHO's ability to make such recommendations flows from its role as disseminator of 'best practices' for public health authorities at the national level.

The IHR and HIV/AIDS examples indicate that the Westphalian template did not prevent WHO from making recommendations to its member states about how they should behave with respect to infectious disease problems. In fact, Article 23 of the WHO Constitution states that the World Health Assembly 'shall have the authority to make recommendations to Members with respect to any matter within the competence of the Organization' (WHO, 1948). WHO has made frequent use of its recommendatory powers over the course of its history, preferring to make non-binding recommendations over crafting binding rules of international law (Fidler, 2003a, p. 288).

The power to make recommendations was also playing a significant role in WHO's efforts to revise the IHR prior to the SARS outbreak. WHO (2002d, p. 9) argued that the revised IHR should authorize WHO to issue recommendations for public health emergencies of international concern. WHO proposed that the revised IHR contain a non-exhaustive list of types of potential recommendations (see Table 7.1). WHO (2002d, p. 9) envisioned the following process for the issuance of recommendations: 'When there is imminent risk of international spread of disease or disruption of international travel and trade, WHO would issue recommendations for action by Member States. These recommendations could be directed at the affected country (containment and control measures), at other Member States, or at both.' The proposed process would involve consultations with the countries potentially affected by such recommendations: 'During an actual public health emergency of international concern, WHO and the concerned State(s) would choose the appropriate measures to be taken from the complete list, and use this as a basis for recommendations for use by Member States' (WHO, 2002d, p. 10).

Table 7.1 Examples of draft measures potentially available for use in a WHO recommendation under the revised IHR

Draft measures potentially applicable at point of entry into non-affected member states from an affected member state
1. **To travelers** -no measures required -require travel history in affected country -require proof of medical examination -require medical examination on entry -require proof of vaccination or other prophylaxis for entry -require vaccination or other prophylaxis for entry -require protective measures for suspected cases -require active or passive medical surveillance from travelers from affected area -require isolation of traveler for incubation period of disease -refuse entry of persons from affected area
2. **To goods and conveyances** -no measures required -require inspection of conveyance, cargo or goods -require treament of conveyance, cargo or goods -require isolation of conveyance, cargo or goods -require destruction of cargo or goods -refuse entry of conveyance, cargo or goods

Source: WHO 2002d, pp. 9–10

These proposals for WHO issuance of recommendations in the revised IHR show WHO attempting to retrofit the Westphalian template for public health governance. WHO had moved toward global health governance with the proposal to incorporate non-governmental sources of information into surveillance; but, as illustrated by the process of WHO and concerned member states jointly deciding what measures would form the basis for recommendations WHO would issue, sovereignty still loomed large with this aspect of the IHR revision. The process described by the WHO does not, in any way, suggest that WHO will or should possess authority under the revised IHR to issue recommendations independently, without the joint participation of the sovereign states directly affected. The revised IHR describe a recommendation process very much beholden to Westphalian sovereignty.

What happened in the SARS outbreak bears no resemblance to what WHO was proposing for the revised IHR. The SARS crisis witnessed WHO acting well beyond the authority it was proposing to write into the revised IHR. The radical nature of WHO's behavior in the SARS epidemic appears in both the substance of the recommendations issued and the process through which WHO issued them. Substantively, the most radical of all the WHO recommendations – the geographically-specific travel advisories – were directed at travelers not WHO member states. For the revised IHR, WHO (2002d, p. 9) proposed that it would issue 'recommendations for action by Member States.' WHO's geographically specific travel advisories during SARS were recommendations not directed at member states but at travelers, non-state actors.

For example, WHO's first geographically-specific travel advisory against Hong Kong and Guangdong Province recommended 'that persons travelling to Hong Kong Special Administrative Region and Guangdong Province, China consider postponing all but essential travel' (WHO, 2003a-1). Subsequent geographically-specific travel advisories followed the same pattern – advising individuals not to travel rather than recommending to WHO member states that they recommend that their nationals postpone all but essential travel.

Although such recommendations can be seen as indirect suggestions that WHO member states take action to reduce travel by their nationals to the SARS-affected areas targeted, the rendering of advice by WHO directly to individual travelers is substantively significant because WHO connects, through such recommendations, with non-state actors directly rather than through the intermediary of the sovereign state. This connection parallels the direct incorporation of non-state actors in the process of gathering global surveillance on infectious diseases. The SARS outbreak finds WHO engaged in both governance input and output directly with non-state actors in a manner that cannot be explained by Westphalian public health.

The geographically-specific travel advisories are also substantively distinct from what WHO was proposing for the revised IHR in another important respect. WHO's list of possible measures that could form the basis for WHO recommendations in the context of a public health emergency of international concern does not include recommendations directly to travelers to postpone non-essential travel to disease-infected areas (see Table 7.1). Although WHO cautioned that its list was non-exhaustive, advising people to postpone travel to certain areas because of health threats was not an alien idea before SARS.

The idea does not appear on WHO's list because the recommendations element of the revised IHR was hewing to the Westphalian emphasis on sovereignty. Getting a country affected by a public health emergency of international concern to agree that WHO should recommend that other countries cut off non-essential travel to it was not realistic. The measures WHO listed would form the basis of recommendations to WHO member states on how to deal with travelers, goods, and conveyances coming from, not going to, disease-affected areas. Yet, in the SARS outbreak, WHO issued numerous recommendations that non-essential travel to certain SARS-affected countries and regions be postponed. Such recommendations go beyond what WHO was contemplating even with the revised IHR.

Equally, and perhaps more, radical than the substantive content of WHO's recommendations was the nature of the process through which WHO issued them. WHO issued all its major alerts and travel advisories without reaching consensus on these actions with the states concerned and often without even consulting with the states directly affected. States subject to a geographically-specific travel advisory from WHO expressed their unhappiness and sometimes outrage at WHO's actions, demonstrating that WHO did not issue such recommendations after consulting and reaching consensus with these states.

The example of the WHO travel advisory issued against Toronto provides an excellent illustration of the process through which WHO issued these travel advisories. WHO issued its Toronto advisory without consulting the Canadian government. Officials at Health Canada 'complained that WHO officials did not give them warning' of the travel advisory (Brown, 2003a), which was 'an absolute stunner,' (National Advisory Committee, 2003, p. 37), leaving Canadian officials fuming at being 'sandbagged' by WHO (Brown and Connolly, 2003).

As noted above, WHO's ideas for the revised IHR included the issuance of recommendations only after consultation with affected states and only jointly with the consent of affected states. During the SARS outbreak, these Westphalian acknowledgements of sovereignty disappear as WHO acted independently. Analyzing WHO's decision to issue its 15 March emergency travel advisory, the *Los Angeles Times* noted that WHO officials 'agonized over how to limit economic damage but concluded that the conservative course – consulting with national governments – had already failed' (Piller, 2003). This observation captures the abandonment of the Westphalian model by WHO during the SARS crisis.

This radical break with established patterns of behavior for an international health organization took place in the context of actions against important states in the international system, especially Canada and China. The action by the WHO Director-General in 1970 to report the cholera outbreak in Guinea without information from the Guinean government (discussed in Chapter 4) represents a much less radical departure from established behavior for two reasons. First, the WHO Director-General took the action against a weak, developing country not a rich nation, such as Canada, or a rising great power, such as China.

Second, the WHO Director-General was attempting to address a clear violation of Guinea's obligation under the IHR to report cholera outbreaks. The IHR were irrelevant to the SARS outbreak, and WHO member states were under no international legal obligations directly addressing this epidemic. Under Westphalian public health, international health organizations should be at their most cautious with, and deferential toward, sovereignty of the member states when such states have not established an international legal framework for dealing with a problem. WHO's boldness and lack of deference for sovereignty during the SARS outbreak is a sign of post-Westphalian public health governance.

The reader should also keep in mind that WHO exercised real power when it issued its geographically-specific travel advisories because these advisories adversely affected the economies of the targeted countries, regions, or cities. As a general matter, international organizations do not exercise independent power because their member states tightly constrain what the organizations can and cannot do. States have certainly never given any international health organization the express or implied power to harm materially the economies of its members during infectious disease outbreaks. The traditional approach has been the creation of international legal disciplines on member states to regulate their actions during outbreaks (e.g., the IHR) not to authorize the international health organization to act without consultation and consensus with its member states.

In issuing alerts and advisories, WHO exercised significant power in the absence of any agreed policy or legal framework and without deference to the sovereignty of affected states. These actions revealed WHO as an autonomous actor influencing events directly rather than just acting as a convenient device for coordinating the sovereign behavior of its member states. Without any express policy or legal basis for its actions, WHO took steps with serious political and economic consequences for states affected by SARS. Again, the Westphalian model of international relations cannot explain this type of behavior by an international organization. WHO's actions signal the emergence of a radically transformed governance context for infectious disease control.

Further evidence of this sea change came in the acquiescence of WHO member states affected by the alerts and advisories to their issuance by WHO. Although targeted countries bristled and bellowed about the travel advisories, none publicly challenged WHO's authority to issue such advisories without their consent. Even Canada, which complained bitterly and lobbied extensively for WHO to lift its travel advisory against Toronto, only challenged whether an advisory was warranted for Toronto rather than attacking the notion that WHO could take such powerful actions without consulting Canada. Officials in China and Taiwan similarly criticized the WHO travel advisories against their territories but did not publicly question whether WHO had the authority to issue such advisories without the participation of the countries being targeted. The widespread acquiescence of sovereign states to the aggregation of power by the WHO in the absence of any express policy or legal framework is astonishing.

Acquiescence turned to formal approval at the May 2003 World Health Assembly meeting, at which the World Health Assembly approved WHO's ability to issue alerts. The World Health Assembly (2003b) asked the WHO Director-General 'to alert, when necessary and after informing the government concerned, the international community to the presence of a public health threat that may constitute a serious threat to neighbouring countries or to international health on the basis of criteria and procedures jointly developed with Members.' In this resolution, the World Health Assembly went beyond the recommendatory powers in WHO's proposals for the revised IHR. The IHR revision proposal sought to create a process where WHO and affected states would jointly choose the appropriate recommendations. The World Health Assembly resolution empowers WHO to issue alerts after merely informing the governments concerned. The resolution limits joint participation of the member states to the development of the criteria and procedures for the exercise of this alert power.

The World Health Assembly's decision is significant for global health governance on infectious diseases. As the SARS outbreak demonstrated, WHO-issued alerts and advisories could cause economic damage by adversely affecting commerce and travel. In contrast to WHO's relative powerlessness in the Westphalian model, WHO now possesses independent authority that carries real power, which WHO members have expressly approved. In the words of one infectious disease specialist at the US Centers for Disease Control and Prevention, WHO 'has assumed "police" powers for controlling outbreaks that put it above national governments, the traditional guardians of public health' (Piller, 2003).

The authority to issue global alerts and advisories connects with the ability to use information from non-governmental sources. WHO member states approved the Organization's ability to issue alerts against sovereign states without their consent based on information collected from governmental and non-governmental sources. Faced with the impossibility of preventing disease information from flowing to the international community, and with the possibility of facing the adverse consequences of a WHO alert based on global surveillance data, a country's incentive to hide an outbreak for fear of the economic consequences has diminished significantly.

The argument that WHO alerts will deter countries from reporting outbreak information (National Intelligence Council, 2003, p. 23) neglects to recall the effect of WHO's ability to collect such information from non-governmental sources. The powers to use non-governmental information and to issue global alerts create a global health governance pincer that squeezes the state's sovereign decision of whether to report outbreak information and to cooperate with WHO and other countries (see Figure 7.2). This pincer changes the way in which states exercise their sovereignty in the context of infectious disease outbreaks and represents evidence of public health's transition into a post-Westphalian governance framework.

Another reflection of public health's arrival in post-Westphalian territory is the subordination of international law witnessed in the handling of the SARS outbreak. States structured Westphalian public health through formal agreements under international law. The IHR serve as the best illustration of this Westphalian approach. The strengthening of global health governance in the wake of the SARS outbreak occurred without any changes in international law on infectious disease control. When SARS emerged, WHO was only in the process of formulating approaches for the revision of the IHR. Formal adoption of the revised IHR was still years away. Although WHO intends to complete the IHR revision process by 2005, the revised IHR will merely reflect changes in infectious disease governance effected before and during the SARS outbreak without the direct use of international law. Rather than being a primary instrument

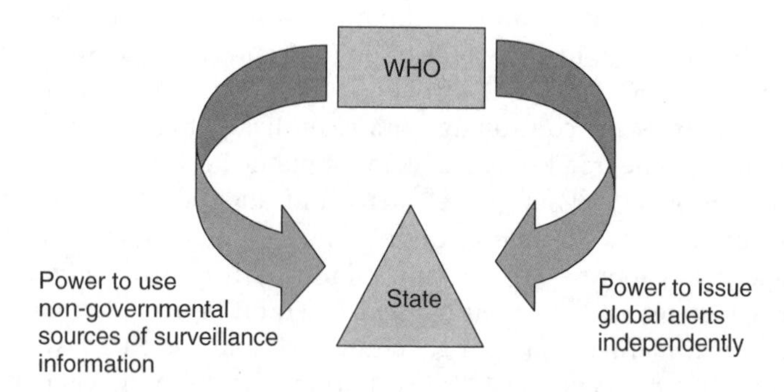

Figure 7.2 The global health governance pincer

used by states to shape future governance, international law has become a secondary mechanism to reflect policy transformations with serious impact on sovereignty that have already taken place.

The SARS outbreak has also produced strengthening of global health governance in the form of a new WHO initiative – the formation of a public–private partnership 'to fight SARS and build capacity for surveillance, epidemiology and public health laboratory facilities in China and the surrounding region' (WHO, 2003c-3). WHO plans to collaborate with the Global Health Initiative of the World Economic Forum to raise $100 million from the global business community, especially enterprises operating in Asia, which monies will fund improvements of surveillance and response capabilities at country-level (WHO, 2003c-3). Nothing equivalent ever appeared under Westphalian public health. As WHO's Executive Director of Communicable Diseases stated, '[t]here have been no resources for this in the past' (Fuhrmans and Naik, 2003).

The initiative connects to global health governance because it actively seeks participation from non-state actors, in this case companies, to address national public health capabilities and their connection to improved global public health. The new public–private partnership also links with global health governance because companies, not states or international organizations, took the lead in proposing the idea when 'a number of companies approached WHO offering money or other support toward eradicating the [SARS] virus' (Fuhrmans and Naik, 2003). This initiative resonates with the interest in vertical governance strategies prevalent in other global health governance efforts, such as the Global Fund to Fight AIDS, Tuberculosis, and Malaria.

The power of global public goods for health

A second area in which the SARS outbreak supports the argument that public health has entered a post-Westphalian stage involves recognition of the power of the production of global public goods for health (GPGH). The SARS crisis witnessed WHO leading efforts to produce information and knowledge on fighting SARS and to make such information and knowledge globally accessible. The information and knowledge was produced in three areas – surveillance data on SARS cases, information on the best clinical practices for managing SARS patients, and basic scientific knowledge about the causative agent of SARS.

Such SARS-related information and knowledge constituted GPGH because (1) no state could be excluded from their consumption; (2) the consumption of the information or knowledge by one state did not limit consumption by other states; and (3) the consumption of such information and knowledge was important for health purposes across national boundaries and traditional regional groupings. In addition, a strong argument can be made that SARS control itself represents a GPGH.

WHO activities to ensure the global flow of surveillance data on SARS cases around the world, and its use of all sources of epidemiological information in the process, represent a GPGH. Surveillance is a critical component of any strategy to control infectious diseases. The information produced by surveillance efforts leads to the formulation and implementation of appropriate public health interventions. During the SARS outbreak, WHO utilized its Global Network to collect, analyze, and disseminate up-to-date information on the number and location of SARS cases, as well as patterns of international transmission. States, international organizations, and non-state actors in every region of the world had access to WHO's SARS surveillance information through WHO's web site. Such non-excludable, non-rival access contributed positively to international and national public health efforts taken to control SARS.

SARS also triggered unprecedented efforts by WHO to make clinical information and experience on managing SARS patients globally available. As discussed in Chapter 5, WHO organized electronic 'grand rounds' through which clinicians handling SARS cases around the world could share information and learn from one another in an effort to construct 'best clinical practices' for SARS case management. As with the global surveillance data WHO produced, the clinical information was also globally accessible and non-excludable and non-rival in its consumption. The absence of adequate diagnostic technologies, drug therapies, and vaccines made such clinical information more important in the global campaign to control SARS.

WHO also coordinated unprecedented global scientific cooperation to generate basic scientific knowledge about the causative agent behind SARS. WHO constructed a network of scientific laboratories stretching around the globe to work synergistically to identify as rapidly as possible the causative pathogen of SARS. Many commentators marveled at the speed, efficiency, and cooperation with which this network identified a new coronavirus (SARS-CoV) as the pathogen responsible for SARS. Julie Gerberding (2003, p. 2030), Director of the US Centers for Disease Control and Prevention, asserted that the '[s]peed of scientific discovery and speed of communication are hallmarks of the response to SARS and reflect amazing achievements in science, technology, and international collaboration.' In this effort, scientific activities on a germ did not recognize borders for the benefit of producing globally useful and needed scientific knowledge.

The scientific information produced by this network remained, by and large, globally accessible to scientific researchers in order to promote the rapid development of diagnostic technologies and possible strategies for a SARS vaccine. The basic scientific knowledge generated about SARS represented a GPGH produced through WHO leadership. Key participants in the global scientific endeavor, such as the US Centers for Disease Control and Prevention, adopted strategies to ensure that knowledge and research techniques developed in the SARS investigation remained publicly available and not subject to private appropriation through intellectual property rights ('SARS: Race to Patent,' 2003). With important scientific information on SARS in the public domain, prospects for the development of effective diagnostic, therapeutic, and prevention technologies as GPGH were enhanced.

The surveillance, clinical, and basic scientific research examples meld together to support the argument that SARS control itself represented a GPGH. As the spread of SARS illustrates, the disease had global scope because of the contribution of air transportation to the spread of SARS-CoV. Unlike other acute respiratory infections, SARS was not primarily a disease of poverty, as evidenced by the damage it caused in affluent societies such as Singapore, Hong Kong, and Canada. With no effective diagnostics, therapies, or prevention technologies, SARS represented a serious global public health threat, especially given its high fatality rate. As a result, control of SARS can be considered a GPGH, as well as the inputs needed to make such control possible (e.g., global surveillance data, effective clinical practices, and basic scientific knowledge concerning the causative pathogen).

More broadly, the SARS outbreak provides support for seeing policy utility in the GPGH concept and for using this concept in the infectious disease control context. Literature on GPGH has analyzed the extent to which control of infectious disease epidemics can be considered a GPGH (Woodward and Smith, 2003; Giesecke, 2003), and part of the discourse concentrates on determining the profile of epidemics the control of which would represent a GPGH. Woodward and Smith (2003, pp. 24–5) argue, for example, that control of HIV/AIDS and tuberculosis can be considered GPGH but control of malaria, acute respiratory infections, diarrheal diseases, and non-eradicable vaccine-preventable diseases are not GPGH.

The SARS outbreak provides an excellent illustration of an epidemic the control of which does represent a GPGH. Infectious diseases with global scope and efficient cross-border transmissibility for which public health authorities have few, if any, technological defenses require different governance approaches than other diseases with other epidemic profiles. With diseases such as SARS, the need for global health governance mechanisms and the production of GPGH, such as global epidemiological, clinical, and scientific data, are heightened as a policy matter. In other words, diseases the control of which constitutes a GPGH represent core territory for post-Westphalian public health.

Elevating public health as a national political priority

A lament of public health officials for decades has been the neglect of public health by governments. In the Westphalian system of international politics, public health was a low priority of states nationally and internationally. When public health became a matter of political concern in the Westphalian system, the driving force was the self-interest of great powers worried about their vulnerability to disease importation and the impact of other nations' health measures on their trade.

Part of the effort to highlight emerging and re-emerging infectious diseases as threats in the 1990s and early 2000s was to increase political attention on public health, particularly to get governments to confront the inadequacies of national and international public health capabilities. Two different tracks are discernable in these various attempts to elevate the political profile of infectious disease control. The first track emphasized the impact of globalization on infectious disease control in order to communicate that the nature of public health governance was being transformed. This track sought to get states to re-think the relationship between sovereignty and public health in light of the globalized reality of pathogenic threats.

The second track attempted to fit the threat from emerging and re-emerging infectious diseases into the traditional great-power model of Westphalian public health. The best example coming from this approach were the arguments made by experts and some government officials that emerging and re-emerging infectious diseases, especially HIV/AIDS, and the threat of bioterrorism constituted a threat to the national security of states, including the great powers. Most of the literature linking infectious disease control and national security focused on the United States, the world's political, military, and economic hegemon. (For more on these arguments, see Chapter 8.)

Before the SARS outbreak, bioterrorism provided the most traction for elevating public health as a political priority, particularly after the anthrax attacks in October 2001 in the United States. The bioterrorism framework fit, however, tightly into the Westphalian pattern of great-power interest driving the direction of public health. Public health officials tried to stress the synergies between bioterrorism preparedness efforts and public health capabilities needed to deal with naturally occurring infectious diseases spread through globalization. Conceptually, the synergies worked in two directions: bioterrorism preparedness benefited public health generally, and general public health improvements benefited bioterrorism preparedness. Before SARS, the lion's share of attention focused on how bioterrorism programs would produce positive externalities for public health, and on how public health improvements would benefit bioterrorism defenses.

The following provides a good example of these American-centric, bioterrorism-driven synergy arguments:

> But a complete strategy against bioterrorism cannot stop at the water's edge. Disease knows no borders, and simply investing in the domestic health system will leave Americans exposed to deadly microbes from abroad. Outside the United States, the public health infrastructure that treats the natural propagation of disease is the same infrastructure that detects, and responds to, diseases that are intentionally spread. This point is critical. An investment in service delivery in other countries is an investment in surveillance and detection on a global scale. This, in turn, reinforces defenses against biological terrorism, while having the added benefit of preventing improper healthcare abroad, which creates strains resistant to modern medicine. (Campbell and Zelikow, 2003, p. 4)

The SARS outbreak has given efforts to elevate public health as a national political priority under the 'globalization track' new momentum. In a globalized world, states need to give public health more attention and resources. Such political concern for public health can play a significant role in addressing threats from globalizing diseases. Reflecting on the SARS crisis, WHO observed that '[o]ne of the most important lessons learned to date is the decisive power of high-level political commitment to contain an outbreak even when sophisticated control tools are lacking' (WHO, 2003t-2). The need for such political commitment cut across the spectrum of states in the international system, implicating rich and poor countries, liberal states and authoritarian regimes. The US National Intelligence Council (2003, p. 29) observed that 'SARS has demonstrated to even skeptical government leaders that health matters in profound social, economic, and political ways.'

SARS also encouraged the elevation of public health as a political priority by demonstrating the economic damage that emerging and re-emerging infectious diseases can cause. States seriously affected by SARS suffered significant economic losses as outbreaks disrupted patterns of commerce and travel and caused feat in the international business community. The SARS outbreak encouraged political leaders to see the capability to detect disease events early, to cooperate with other nations, and to intervene swiftly and effectively as key components of *economic* policy in the era of globalization.

Viewing the connection between infectious disease control and economic policy in this fashion suggests the emergence of post-Westphalian public health. The Westphalian connection between public health and economic policy flowed from the great powers' interest in reducing the trade impact of other nations' infectious-disease control measures (e.g., maritime quarantine). The great powers' economic interest in infectious disease control did not extend into their own capabilities to manage infectious disease outbreaks largely because domestic public health improvements in these countries reduced the vulnerability of the great powers to disease importation.

As SARS demonstrates, the post-Westphalian context finds great powers and weak countries confronted with an *economic need* to improve the public health capabilities of managing globalized microbial traffic. This need translates not into strategies of self-help, as the great powers adopted in the Westphalian period, but into recognition of the role for global health governance and the production of GPGH, as is happening in the post-Westphalian period. Even the United States under the unilateralist-minded Bush administration did not, despite rumblings of misgivings, oppose WHO's revolutionary actions during the SARS outbreak and their subsequent approval by the World Health Assembly as the framework for future epidemic management.

The post-Westphalian context for infectious disease control also encourages public health's elevation as a political priority. As China discovered to its embarrassment, WHO's ability to use non-governmental sources of surveillance information revealed serious weaknesses in China's systems of public health and health care delivery. Such weakened health infrastructure contributed to SARS' spread in China and the eventual economic damage China suffered from becoming a SARS 'hot zone.' The recipe for avoiding global humiliation and economic damage in the context of a post-Westphalian outbreak calls for upgrading of public health and health care capabilities. Less dramatically, other countries, such as Canada and Taiwan, felt the global political and economic pain of allowing a new infectious disease to gain a foothold in their territories. In the aftermath of such pain, public health and health care infrastructures can no longer be considered secondary priorities for governments confronted with managing globalized anarchy. Canada's National Advisory Committee on SARS and Public Health emphasized the political importance of public health in the post-SARS world by recalling Benjamin Disraeli's argument that 'public health was the foundation for "the happiness of the people and the power of the country. The care of the public health is the first duty of the statesman"' (National Advisory Committee, 2003, p. 220).

Reinforcing the public health–human rights linkage

The SARS outbreak highlights a fourth area that points toward the emergence of a post-Westphalian period for public health – the role of human rights in public health policy. Under Westphalian public health, human rights did not register as a concern because states were considered the only legitimate actors for purposes of governance. Further, the principles of sovereignty and non-intervention created significant barriers for the development of human rights as an element of international health governance. The human rights movement began to challenge Westphalian public health in the aftermath of World War II, as illustrated by the statement in the preamble of the WHO Constitution that the right to the highest attainable standard of health is a fundamental human right (WHO, 1948).

Still, the relationship between public health and human rights took a long time to gain attention, which began to happen in the late 1970s through the Health for All movement (Declaration of Alma Ata, 1978). The public health–human rights linkage became more prominent after HIV/AIDS exploded on the world. As discussed in Chapter 4, HIV/AIDS caused public health communities to turn to international human rights law to help guide policy on the epidemic because traditional approaches to infectious disease governance (e.g., the IHR) lacked utility.

This public health turn toward human rights brought both civil and political rights (e.g., freedom of movement) and economic, social, and cultural rights (e.g., the right to health) to bear on public health. Civil and political rights became a policy instrument in the fight against stigma and discrimination faced by people living with HIV/AIDS. The right to health became a weapon in advocacy for greater access to primary health care services and essential medicines, including anti-retrovirals. HIV/AIDS led public health away from the traditional, state-centric Westphalian approaches to infectious diseases toward a strategy that placed individuals and their rights, not states and their sovereignty, at the center of concern.

The SARS outbreak reinforces this post-Westphalian move toward the public health–human rights linkage but in ways different from what occurred with HIV/AIDS. The widespread resort by countries to isolation and quarantine, and the recommendations of WHO to use these public health instruments, brought to life concerns about public health measures infringing civil and political rights, such as freedom of movement (McNeil, 2003; Fidler, 2003b). Treaties protecting civil and political rights have long recognized public health as a legitimate reason for infringing on certain individual rights (Fidler, 1999, pp. 172–3).

However, apart from human rights criticisms of isolation and quarantine as responses to HIV/AIDS and concern about compulsory treatment of individuals infected with multi-drug resistant tuberculosis, striking the proper balance between the protection of population health and respect for civil and political rights has not been a prominent question for public health policy in the post-World War II era mainly because quarantine and isolation largely disappeared from public health practice. The proper balance between public health and individual liberties became a matter of prominent debate in the late 1990s and early 2000s in the context of the development of US bioterrorism policy (Annas, 2002), but this debate largely took place within the framework of US constitutional jurisprudence rather than international law on human rights.

The SARS outbreak made the question of balancing the protection of public health and respect for individual rights a pressing concern, which represents yet another governance deviation from the Westphalian model. In the HIV/AIDS context, public health officials and human rights activists used international human rights law to restrain the power and indifference of the state vis-à-vis individuals living with HIV/AIDS. SARS produced a different focus: At times, governments may need to infringe on civil and political rights in order to deal with an infectious disease.

The different policy responses of governments affected by SARS indicate that the question of the proper balance between public health and individual rights received different answers. In some countries, such as Singapore, the government used compulsory and tightly monitored isolation and quarantine (Pottinger, 2003d), thus producing significant infringements on civil and political rights. Other countries, such as Canada, relied more on voluntary isolation and quarantine strategies than on compulsory powers (McNeil, 2003), creating an approach with less adverse impact on individual rights. And still other nations, such as the United States, did not use voluntary quarantine in cases where other countries utilized compulsory or voluntary quarantine (e.g., with respect to individuals who were in contact with suspect SARS cases) (US CDC, 2003).

These varying approaches to balancing public health and human rights mean that SARS creates the need for further examination and application of the criteria international human rights law establishes to evaluate public health measures that infringe on civil and political rights. The criteria are four and derive from the application of the Siracusa Principles on the Limitations and Derogation Provisions in the International Covenant on Civil and Political Rights (Siracusa, 1985): The rights-infringing measure must (1) be prescribed by law; (2) be applied in a non-discriminatory manner; (3) relate to a compelling public interest in the form of a significant risk to the public's health; and (4) be necessary to achieve the protection of the public, meaning that the measure must be (a) based on scientific and public health information and principles; (b) proportional in its impact on individual rights to the threat posed; and (c) the least restrictive measure possible to achieve protection against the infectious disease risk.

In terms of determining whether an individual with an infectious disease poses a significant risk to the public's health, four factors are important: (1) the nature of the infectious disease risk, including the mode of transmission of the infectious agent; (2) the duration of the infectious disease risk, including how long the individual is capable of transmitting the infectious agent; (3) the probability that the individual will transmit the disease, which involves evaluating how the infectious disease is transmitted and how often such transmission acts are likely to occur; and (4) the severity of the consequences if the individual does transmit the infectious disease.

With these criteria and factors in mind, a strong case can be made that isolation and quarantine with respect to SARS cases and suspect cases was warranted under international human rights law. Most governments have enacted public health statutes that authorize isolation and quarantine as measures to control infectious diseases, even if many of these statutes are old and have not been used in decades. Some countries, such as the United States, revised their laws in 2003 to be able to deal directly with SARS (US Public Health Service Act, 2003). Thus, the requirement that rights-restricting measures be prescribed by law was, in most cases, readily satisfied.

Isolation and quarantine measures for SARS can also be seen as relating to a compelling public interest in the form of a significant infectious disease threat. SARS is caused by a novel virus about which little is known, transmitted from person-to-person by respiratory means, and is fatal in a relatively high percentage of cases (e.g., 14–15 per cent fatality rate). Further, no adequate diagnostic technologies or anti-viral therapies exist to help manage the disease. Thus, SARS qualifies as a significant threat to public health under international human rights law.

The use of isolation and quarantine to control SARS can also be considered to be based on scientific and public health information and principles, proportional in its impact on individual rights to the threat SARS poses to public health, and the least restrictive measures possible to achieve protection against the spread of the disease. These conclusions largely flow from the serious threat SARS poses as a contagious disease and the absence of any diagnostic, therapeutic, and prevention technologies that could be used to mitigate the infringement on civil and political rights. SARS-related isolation and control measures also do not appear to have been characterized by their discriminatory application by governments in SARS-affected countries.

This cursory analysis of the use of isolation and quarantine during the SARS outbreak does not mean that all isolation and quarantine measures enacted, or that could be enacted, to deal with SARS were or will be necessarily permissible under international human rights law. The diverse approaches of countries to isolation and quarantine during the SARS outbreak raises the need to evaluate the appropriateness of such measures to deal with this disease, even when isolation and quarantine for SARS appear reasonable in a quick review of the criteria and factors embedded in international human rights law.

With public health experts warning that SARS may return and even become endemic, isolation and quarantine may remain key public health instruments until more effective public health strategies involving diagnostic, therapeutic, and prevention technologies develop. Additionally, the global health governance pincer formed by the ability to use non-governmental sources of surveillance information and the authority to issue economically damaging global alerts may encourage governments to resort more rapidly and frequently to isolation and quarantine in order to ensure that the pincer is kept at bay, even when isolation and quarantine may not in fact be warranted. For example, once China decided to respond seriously to SARS, its SARS-control efforts involved 'the application of very draconian measures' (Pei, 2003). For a host of reasons, the SARS outbreak invites more rigorous attention to be paid to the human rights implications of isolation and quarantine as part of the post-Westphalian governance context for public health.

All's well that ends well?

This chapter analyzed four features of the SARS outbreak that confirm public health's transition into a post-Westphalian environment. These features underscore and expand the lessons learned from China's mishandling of SARS examined in Chapter 6. The proposition that SARS represents the world's first post-Westphalian pathogen is compelling in light of what happened in the SARS outbreak both within and beyond China. Compared with the depressing advance of pathogenic microbes over the last few decades, and the seeming inability of existing governance structures to address this advance effectively, the successful governance response to SARS stands out as a beacon of hope in humanity's ongoing struggle with infectious diseases.

But, as the next chapter explores, the successful ending of the global SARS effort and the transition into post-Westphalian governance does not necessarily mean that all is well in public health's 'new world order.'

8
SARS and Vulnerabilities of Post-Westphalian Public Health

The other side of the Rubicon

Reflecting on the experience of handling the SARS epidemic, WHO's Mike Ryan observed that '[a] Rubicon has been crossed. There's no going back now' (Piller, 2003). As previous chapters illuminated, the SARS outbreak confirms that public health has moved into post-Westphalian governance territory with respect to infectious diseases. The successful management of the global SARS threat provides ample evidence that the governance possibilities in post-Westphalian public health possess exciting potential. Much future work, including the completion of the revision of the International Health Regulations and the establishment of the public–private partnership to fund improvements in national SARS-related surveillance and response capabilities, will focus on exploiting the possibilities revealed dramatically in the SARS crisis.

At the same time, the other side of the Rubicon public health crossed during the SARS outbreak deserves more critical attention. In addition to highlighting the shift from Westphalian to post-Westphalian public health, the SARS epidemic contains features that suggest that post-Westphalian public health faces vulnerabilities that may erode some of the promise now seen in the strategies used to respond and contain SARS in 2003. This chapter examines some of the governance problems that post-Westphalian public health confronts in the post-SARS environment.

The analysis in this chapter does not, however, constitute predictions about how public health will fare on the other side of the Rubicon. Historic public health accomplishments have, in the past, been followed by the emergence of unexpected public health nightmares. A good example is the emergence of HIV/AIDS immediately after the global triumph of the eradication of smallpox. Similarly, the global crisis of emerging and re-emerging infectious diseases identified in the 1990s dashed notions that modern science had equipped societies to conquer pathogenic microbes. The transition to post-Westphalian governance is not reassuring in every instance involving public health threats because this transition represents the continuation of the struggle to find ways to fend off the relentless pressure created by the interactions of the microbial and human worlds. Public health governance will continue to confront the volatile mixture of germs and politics in the 'new world order' for public health ushered in by the SARS outbreak.

Crossing prior Rubicons: The fate of previous governance innovations in international infectious disease control

What happened in the global campaign to contain SARS was revolutionary from a governance perspective. The SARS outbreak will go down in public health history as a landmark innovation in the handling of international infectious disease problems. Although understanding this innovation on its own terms is important, a broader historical perspective is needed in order to put the governance developments of the SARS crisis into context. Public health governance on infectious disease control has experienced significant innovations in the past, all of which became ineffective over time. Reviewing the fate of these previous governance innovations in the area of infectious diseases should moderate enthusiasm for the potential of the governance revolution witnessed during the SARS epidemic.

The first significant innovation in governance of infectious diseases internationally occurred when public health emerged as a diplomatic issue in the mid-nineteenth century. The diplomatic emergence of infectious diseases as a foreign policy issue marked a significant change in the nature of the Westphalian system of public health governance. As discussed in Chapter 3, prior to the convening of the first International Sanitary Conference in 1851, governance of infectious diseases was national in orientation. The elevation of infectious disease control to the subject of diplomatic activity in the mid-nineteenth century created new governance activities at the intergovernmental level. The governance innovations spawned by this new approach to infectious disease problems included the periodic international sanitary conferences and international sanitary conventions through which states sought to achieve international governance on infectious disease threats.

Not long after the elevation of infectious disease control to a foreign policy concern, experts and officials working the new machinery of international health governance realized that the innovations of ad hoc diplomatic conferences and the negotiation of different international sanitary conventions were inadequate governance responses to the infectious disease problem. The nature of the threat posed by pathogenic microbes in an increasingly interdependent world forced the developing framework of Westphalian public health to undergo revision. States reformed the Westphalian approach through another governance innovation – the creation of permanent international health organizations charged with overseeing the international sanitary conventions and/or coordinating intergovernmental cooperation on infectious diseases. Through these reforms Westphalian public health governance became more centralized at the intergovernmental level.

In time, these reforms to the Westphalian model also proved inadequate in addressing the threat posed by pathogenic microbes. The next governance reforms appeared in four areas: (1) the consolidation of the various international health organizations into one universal organization, WHO; (2) the creation of a different process for crafting international legal rules on infectious diseases in the form of the adoption of international regulations under Articles 21 and 22 of the WHO Constitution; (3) the unification of international legal rules on infectious disease control to provide one set of rules for the international community, the International Health Regulations; and (4) articulating infectious disease control as part of the individual human right to the highest attainable standard of health.

The first two decades of the twentieth century witnessed the creation of three different international health organizations – the Pan American Sanitary Bureau (1902), the *Office International de l'Hygiène Publique* (1907), and the Health Organization of the League of Nations (1923). Despite efforts to coordinate the activities of these various bodies, the existence of multiple entities created inefficiencies and frictions that could only be overcome by consolidating intergovernmental cooperation on public health in one universal organization. The creation of WHO in 1948 as a specialized agency of the United Nations fulfilled this governance need. The first function listed in Article 2 of the WHO Constitution is for the Organization 'to act as the directing and co-ordinating authority on international health work' (WHO, 1948, Article 2(a)), thus giving WHO primacy in terms of intergovernmental cooperation on public health – an organizational primacy that did not exist in prior efforts at international health governance.

The WHO Constitution also addressed another perceived defect in international health governance on infectious diseases – the existence of multiple international sanitary conventions. Experts argued that the many international treaties that existed on infectious disease control created an inefficient, patchwork regime that provided an inadequate framework for addressing the infectious disease threat in international relations. The plethora of treaties produced between 1851 and 1945 made international law on infectious diseases confusing and unsatisfactory by the end of World War II for three reasons.

First, the different treaties created holes in the international regime for infectious disease control. As argued in 1947 by the US Department of State (1947, p. 957), '[t]here are states, including some which occupy key positions in the stream of international maritime and aerial commerce, bound by only the obsolete conventions of 1912, 1926, and 1933, or by no sanitary conventions at all.' Second, the agreements often overlapped in substantive content, were not kept current as scientific knowledge advanced, and were not designed to cope with the increasing speed, volume, and scope of international travel and trade (Fluss, 1997, p. 379). Third, international infectious disease control relied exclusively on the treaty. In connection with infectious disease control, the treaty process proved cumbersome, slow, and resistant to revisions demanded by changing scientific knowledge and patterns of international trade (US Department of State, 1947, p. 957).

The governance innovation created to deal with these problems appears in Articles 21 and 22 of the WHO Constitution (WHO, 1948). Article 21 empowers the World Health Assembly to 'adopt regulations concerning:... sanitary and quarantine requirements and other procedures designed to prevent the international spread of disease.' Article 22 provides that '[r]egulations adopted pursuant to Article 21 shall come into force for all Members after due notice has been given of their adoption by the Health Assembly except for such Members as may notify the Director-General of rejection or reservations within the period stated in the notice.'

As mentioned in Chapter 3, the Article 21–22 combination creates a process different from the normal treaty-making approach. With treaties, states have to 'opt in' – affirmatively declare their willingness to be bound by the rules in the agreements. Article 22 establishes an 'opt out' approach – WHO member states are bound by regulations adopted by the World Health Assembly under Article 21, unless they expressly opt out of the regulations in question.

The governance innovation represented by the Article 21–22 combination was recognized when the WHO was created. Walter Sharp (1947, p. 525) described Article 22 of the WHO Constitution as adopting the 'comparatively novel principle known as 'contracting out'.' Sharp (1947, p. 526) noted that delegations negotiating the WHO Constitution pushed for the innovation in Article 22 to allow WHO to apply new scientific techniques and knowledge efficiently and universally to the international legal rules on infectious diseases. Sharp (1947, p. 525) also observed that Article 22 'was the subject of warm debate' because states worried about the effect of this governance innovation on their sovereignty.

Articles 21 and 22 became the legal basis for the 1951 adoption of the International Sanitary Regulations (1951), the precursor to the International Health Regulations (IHR). With the International Sanitary Regulations, WHO unified the disparate international legal rules scattered across the many international sanitary conventions in existence into a single set of rules for use by WHO member states. WHO, thus, simplified and harmonized the legal framework for international governance for infectious diseases, which represents the third major governance innovation to occur in the immediate post-World War II period.

The IHR also limited the discretion of sovereign states by requiring that all reservations be approved by the World Health Assembly (IHR, 1969, Article 88.1). This provision was designed to deter WHO member states from making reservations to the IHR that would threaten their public health and scientific integrity. The process of having to seek World Health Assembly approval for reservations to the IHR reduced the normal flexibility states had under international law to make reservations to treaties they wished to join. In the IHR, the quasi-legislative powers of Article 21, the 'opt out' technique of Article 22, and subjecting all reservations to acceptance by the World Health Assembly work together, in theory, to provide robust governance for infectious disease control that is not weakened by WHO member states refusing to join or by significant reservations to key provisions.

The fourth major governance innovation to appear in the post-World War II period was the articulation of infectious disease control as part of the individual human right to the highest attainable standard of health. The WHO Constitution contains the first pronouncement that the enjoyment of the highest attainable standard of health was a fundamental human right (WHO, 1948, Preamble). Later international legal instruments, such as the International Covenant on Economic, Cultural, and Social Rights (ICESCR), also proclaimed the enjoyment of the highest attainable standard of health a human right (ICECSR, 1966, Article 12). Part of the responsibility of states under the right to health included the prevention, treatment, and control of epidemic and endemic diseases, including infectious diseases (ICESCR, 1966, Article 12.2(c)). Framing infectious disease control in the context of the fulfillment of a fundamental human right represented a governance innovation because it identified individuals, not just states, as subjects of international law on infectious diseases.

The crisis in emerging and re-emerging infectious diseases identified in the 1990s and early 2000s revealed the extent to which public health experts were dissatisfied with each of these four governance innovations. By the mid-1990s, WHO's ability to act as the directing and coordinating authority on international health work was questioned and under attack (Godlee, 1994a; Godlee, 1994b; Godlee, 1997). Other international organizations not expressly dedicated to public health, such as the World Bank, International Monetary Fund, and the World Trade Organization, were increasingly seen by experts as more powerful and important players in public health than WHO. As one WHO official put it, '[t]he World Bank is the new 800-pound gorilla in world health care' (Abbassi, 1999, p. 865).

The IHR's collapse as an international legal regime on infectious disease control (analyzed in Chapter 3) suggested that the governance reforms of unifying international law on infectious diseases and the 'opt out' process had little, if any, impact. The human right to health similarly appeared to carry little influence with WHO member states in terms of infectious disease control, a reality confirmed by the growing toll infectious diseases, especially HIV/AIDS, were causing around the world as the twentieth century drew to a close. Katarina Tomasevski (1995, p. 873) captured the stagnation into which the human right to health had fallen by the mid-1990s when she argued that 'the right to health has not conceptually progressed from the time it was first proclaimed, not even to define the core terms *health* and *right* in the proclaimed right to health.'

A comprehensive analysis of why these previous governance innovations led to dissatisfaction in the world of public health is beyond the scope of this chapter, but some general observations are in order. First, three of the four governance reforms described above represent reforms from within the Westphalian governance framework. The creation of a single international health organization with primacy on international health work, the quasi-legislative authority of the World Health Assembly to adopt international regulations through the 'opt out' procedure, and the unification of international law on infectious diseases in the IHR remained firmly within the template of Westphalian governance. Only the linkage between infectious disease control and the human right to health moved beyond the Westphalian model by incorporating individuals as formal subjects of international law. As governance responses to emerging and re-emerging infectious diseases in the 1990s and early 2000s (analyzed in Chapter 4) suggested, the main problem was the Westphalian template. Tinkering with the template did not significantly improve infectious disease control.

Second, the promise initially sensed with each of the four governance reforms described above never panned out for two basic reasons: (1) the commitment of governments to public health nationally and internationally waxed and waned, but mainly waned; and (2) political, economic, social, and technological changes created conditions encouraging the emergence and re-emergence of infectious diseases. In short, national and international governance on infectious diseases stagnated while the opportunities for pathogenic microbes to emerge and spread proliferated. The lack of political commitment from governments and globalization's stimulation of the resurgence of infectious diseases led to acknowledgment that the Westphalian approach, and all the reforms made to it, did not provide an adequate governance framework.

The move from a Westphalian to a post-Westphalian approach merely represents the latest attempt at governance innovation in the area of public health generally and infectious disease control specifically. Believing that public health has reached the 'end of history' with respect to governance of infectious diseases in the post-Westphalian period would be naïve in the extreme. The successful handling of the SARS outbreak does not ensure that the commitment of governments to better public health governance has reached a point at which backsliding is impossible. The containment of SARS does not mean that globalization's contributions to microbial incubation, emergence, and spread have waned to the point at which they are easily managed. Previous governance innovations in the area of infectious disease control proved unsustainable, and the sustainability of post-Westphalian public health governance will also be a serious issue that bears close observation.

Rubicons not crossed: The limited applicability of WHO's new global alert power

One danger in focusing too intensely on the SARS outbreak and the governance innovations that sprang from its handling is losing sight of many other global infectious disease problems that exist. The epidemiological profile of SARS – a novel virus communicable through respiratory means for which no diagnostic, therapeutic, or vaccine technologies exist – is not the profile of many of the most serious infectious disease problems facing the world today and in the near future. The relevance of some of the strategies employed in SARS to the governance of other killer diseases is, thus, in doubt.

Much of the governance architecture used in the SARS outbreak does apply to other infectious disease threats, especially the incorporation of non-governmental sources of information into global surveillance, the enhanced response opportunities provided by improved surveillance, and the central role of WHO in global infectious disease surveillance and response. The use by WHO of global alerts and travel advisories is, however, not a governance feature that transfers readily to most of the major infectious disease problems countries face today. Thus, the most jaw-dropping and controversial governance aspect of the containment of SARS will not play a significant role in bringing other epidemic and endemic diseases under control.

The global health governance strategy of incorporating non-governmental sources of information into global surveillance effectively used in the SARS outbreak has general applicability to infectious disease problems. Surveillance is critical to the management of any infectious disease threat. Improvements in the quantity and quality of surveillance information achieved through the collection, analysis, and dissemination of data from both governmental and non-governmental sources are possible across a wide spectrum of infectious diseases. WHO's *Disease Outbreak News* has, from 1996 until the present, posted information on 51 different diseases and syndromes (WHO, 2003d-3), which reflects the broad range of infectious diseases handled by WHO's system of global surveillance, including its Global Outbreak and Alert Response Network (Global Network).

Better surveillance of infectious disease problems creates enhanced opportunities for effective response activities, as illustrated in the handling of the SARS outbreak. Access to improved surveillance data allows national public health authorities to plan and implement control and containment interventions and catalyzes international assistance for countries that need it. Prior to SARS, WHO (2002a, p. 60) noted the link between its surveillance activities and the Global Network when it reported that '[d]uring the past two years, the network has launched broad and effective international containment activities in Afghanistan, Bangladesh, Burkina Faso, Côte d'Ivoire, Egypt, Ethiopia, Gabon, Kosovo, Sierra Leone, Sudan, Uganda, and Yemen. These activities are in addition to many smaller responses requiring technical support or assistance through the provision of vaccines and other supplies.'

The effectiveness of post-Westphalian infectious disease surveillance and response can be seen in examples recorded by WHO with respect to plague in India, Crimean-Congo haemorrhagic fever on the Pakistan–Afghanistan border, relapsing fever in Sudan, and Ebola in Uganda. In each case, early identification of the outbreak through improved surveillance facilitated effective cooperative responses involving national and international public health assets (WHO, 2002a, pp. 65–7). In the examples from India, Sudan, and Uganda, WHO measured the contributions made by the Global Network by comparing the surveillance and response efforts of identical outbreaks in those countries and regions prior to the establishment of the Global Network. In WHO's opinion, the Global Network has made an 'immediate – and measurable – difference' to surveillance and response for infectious diseases (WHO, 2002a, p. 65). WHO calculates the difference the Global Network has made in terms of its ability to address an outbreak without disrupting trade and tourism, by correcting potentially damaging speculation in the news media, by effectively containing the spread of the disease, and by reducing overall morbidity and mortality from the disease (WHO, 2002a, pp. 65–7).

The demands of enhanced surveillance and response activities in a globalized world place a premium on WHO's abilities to manage global flows of epidemiological information and coordinate international assistance for disease control and containment (Grein *et al.*, 2000, p. 97). The need for a strong role for WHO reaches across the spectrum of infectious diseases, from those, such as SARS, that pose global threats to those, such as human African trypanosomiasis, that constitute regional public health problems. Without an effective WHO, the operation of global health governance and the production of global/regional public goods for health would not be possible. This reasoning explains why WHO (2003c-3) is seeking $100 million from 'bilateral donors to support expanded surveillance and response across the globe.' (This $100 million initiative is *in addition* to the $100 million public–private partnership established to fund improvements in SARS-related surveillance and response capabilities in China and the Asian region.)

Although many of the governance features used effectively in the SARS outbreak contribute on a daily basis to WHO's global efforts to identify and contain infectious diseases, the power WHO exercised during the SARS outbreak to issue global alerts and travel advisories is of more limited value in the general fight against pathogenic microbes. As WHO (2003b, p. 3) noted during the SARS crisis, most of the previous outbreaks of new infectious diseases in the decade preceding SARS remained geographically confined because of, among other things, a lack of efficient human-to-human transmission. Not all new diseases that emerge after SARS will share its respiratory transmission capabilities.

Further, governance of three of the major infectious disease killers – HIV/AIDS, tuberculosis, and malaria – is not enhanced, at present, by WHO's ability to issue global alerts and travel warnings. Reflecting on the use of this power in the SARS outbreak, WHO itself 'warned that scourges such as AIDS or malaria will require other approaches and massive new funding' (Piller, 2003). The nature of the Global Fund to Fight AIDS, Tuberculosis, and Malaria demonstrates that governance of these three killer diseases will demand strategies that do not involve WHO issuing global alerts.

The possibility also exists that WHO member states may revisit the issue of whether WHO should issue the kind of global alerts and travel advisories the Organization did during the SARS outbreak. The anger of WHO member states subject to the geographically-specific travel advisories (such as China and Canada) cannot be entirely discounted, even in light of the World Health Assembly's authorization for WHO to issue global alerts when necessary. For example, Health Canada's National Advisory Committee on SARS and Public Health pointedly raised WHO's travel advisory power as a 'discussion point' for further consideration in the aftermath of SARS (National Advisory Committee, 2003, p. 37). The Committee also observed that '[s]ome have suggested that WHO should confine itself to informing countries of the epidemiologic situation in member countries and not issue travel advisories' (National Advisory Committee, 2003, p. 202). Experts within countries affected by the geographically-specific travel advisories have also raised the question of whether the travel advisories made any measurable contribution to the containment of SARS. Paul Gully of Health Canada argued, for example, that it is 'appropriate to look at those travel warnings and ask, "Did it make any difference?"' (Piller, 2003). Another Canadian health official, Allison McGeer, warned that the kind of travel advisories WHO issued during the SARS outbreak are blunt, haphazard tools of unproved effectiveness that need to be assessed to ensure 'they are having positive impact' (Piller, 2003). Canada's National Advisory Committee argued that the criteria WHO used 'seem arbitrary and were developed during the outbreak without a formal consultation process or serious scientific debate,' and the Committee could 'find little rationale for the criteria or the timing of the WHO travel advisory' against Toronto (National Advisory Committee, 2003, p. 203).

The wording of the IHR resolution provides WHO member states concerned about WHO's future use of global alerts and travel advisories some room to place limits on this WHO power. The resolution authorizes the WHO Director-General to issue alerts to the international community 'on the basis of criteria and procedures jointly developed with Member States' (World Health Assembly, 2003b). This language provides concerned WHO member states with the opportunity to circumscribe WHO's alert power by restricting the criteria and procedures under which WHO may exercise the power.

Health Canada's National Advisory Committee on SARS and Public Health recommended, in fact, that Canada should seek to launch a multilateral process that would establish agreed standards of evidence for the issuance of travel advisories and alerts by member states and that would determine 'the role of WHO in issuing travel advice, and to establish a procedure for providing advance notice for possible alerts and advice' (National Advisory Committee, 2003, p. 207). The Committee also recommended that 'the notice process should provide a mechanism for consultation with and a response by the target country' (National Advisory Committee, 2003, p. 207). These recommendations do not seek to strip WHO of the power to issue travel advisories recognized in the World Health Assembly, but they propose a process through which disciplines and limitations on WHO's power would be negotiated and agreed by WHO member states.

I make these observations not to diminish the importance and revolutionary nature of WHO's global alert and travel advisory powers in post-Westphalian public health governance. The use of these powers during SARS, and their subsequent confirmation by the World Health Assembly, constitute very important features of public health's crossing of the post-Westphalian Rubicon during the SARS outbreak. The lack of utility of these powers in the global struggle against major infectious disease threats, such as HIV/AIDS, tuberculosis, malaria, and many neglected infectious diseases that plague only developing countries, highlights the daunting challenges that remain for post-Westphalian public health. Other post-Westphalian Rubicons remain to be crossed, including those represented by the development of safe, effective, and affordable antimicrobial technologies for prevention (e.g., new vaccines) and treatment (e.g., new antimicrobials to address the advance of antimicrobial resistance).

Stagnation after crossing: The sustainability of post-Westphalian governance

Experts reflecting on the national and international efforts made during the SARS outbreak have argued that this outbreak significantly stressed public health capabilities at all levels. There was acknowledgement that no public health system could have sustained effectively its heightened SARS response over a longer period of time simply because of the scale and nature of the threat and the inadequacy of public health resources and assets. These observations were made in connection with SARS-affected countries that were, relatively speaking, equipped with modern public health infrastructures. Sustainability of SARS efforts in countries lacking sophisticated public health capabilities would be even more difficult, if not impossible.

The sustainability concern helps explain why public health experts are very keen to advance the development of effective diagnostics, vaccines, and therapies for SARS. Such technological breakthroughs would provide public health officials with additional weapons and decrease their reliance on isolation and quarantine. Technological breakthroughs would also allow SARS control to proceed in a manner that infringes less on civil rights and liberties.

Likewise, the sustainability of post-Westphalian public health governance dramatically ushered in by the SARS outbreak is not a foregone conclusion. As indicated in an earlier section of this chapter, previous governance innovations lost momentum, influence, and even relevance, becoming stagnant reminders of the failure of political commitment and the relentless pressure microbes create on human societies in globalized times. The epidemiological and political soundness of post-Westphalian forms of public health governance does not make such governance immune from stagnation.

Historically, public health has faced a 'sustainability conundrum.' When infectious diseases pose significant economic and health threats, government commitment to protecting population health typically increases. Subsequent improvements in public health capabilities often lead to decreases in morbidity and mortality associated with infectious diseases. Political interest in public health wanes, leading to complacency and a deterioration of public health capabilities. All this transpires as trade and travel increase rapidly in speed and geographical scope. Stagnation in public health governance leads to new crises with infectious diseases, producing heightened political commitment. The cycle begins again. The conundrum for public health is finding a way to stop success from leading to failure.

Warnings from WHO and other public health organizations and experts about the dangers of complacency with respect to SARS seek to prevent another cycle of the sustainability conundrum with respect to this new disease. More generally, the same warnings need to be issued in connection with the overall post-Westphalian governance architecture. This architecture will not be resilient against the alliance formed between pathogenic microbes and the forces of globalization unless the structure is constantly strengthened, repaired, and enlarged. As Margaret Hamburg (2003, p. 6) argued in testimony to the US House of Representatives, the SARS outbreak teaches that:

> The magnitude and urgency of the problem [of infectious diseases] demand renewed concern and commitment. We have not done enough – in our own defense or in the defense of others. As we take stock of our prospects with respect to microbial threats in the years ahead, we must recognize the need for a new level of attention, dedication, and sustained resources to ensure the health and safety of this nation – and the world.

The historical record does not provide much evidence that post-Westphalian public health will escape the sustainability conundrum. The recognition of the need for a single international organization to direct and coordinate international health work seen in WHO's creation did not prevent states from allowing WHO to lose prestige and effectiveness over the course of its first 50 years. SARS helped underscore WHO's critical role in post-Westphalian public health governance; but this recognition does not automatically equate to sustained interest in, and political and financial support for, the Organization.

The stories of the re-emergence of many infectious diseases, including cholera, yellow fever, malaria, and tuberculosis, are tales of the political and economic neglect of public health nationally, regionally, and internationally. Even post-Westphalian governance initiatives established before SARS face sustainability problems. For example, the sustainability of the Global Fund to Fight AIDS, Tuberculosis, and Malaria has not been assured because, as mentioned in Chapter 4, funding for this new global health governance mechanism remains a serious, ongoing problem. Problems also plague funding of the Roll Back Malaria initiative, a public–private partnership launched in 1998 by WHO to reduce malaria in the developing world, including inadequate pledged donations and failure to disburse pledged donations in full (Narasimhan and Attaran, 2003).

Increasing political and financial support for SARS-control efforts does not necessarily mean that commitment for public health generally has increased. Responses to new problems, such as SARS, may have a parasitic effect on other public health programs because governments merely shift existing funds from one problem to another without actually increasing the size of the overall financial commitment. This shifting effect could have adverse implications for post-Westphalian public health governance. As WHO (2003q-2) indicated in connection with China, '[m]easures may need to be found for sustaining China's present monumental effort to contain SARS, particularly as programmes for responding to other priority diseases, such as HIV/AIDS and TB, may suffer in the long run.' In relation to HIV/AIDS, the US National Intelligence Council (2003, p. 31) argued that 'SARS has focused greater international attention on the importance of health, but the new disease probably will not lead to a significant boost in the fight against HIV/AIDS in the coming years. Indeed, many countries are likely to view spending on diseases like SARS and HIV/AIDS as a zero-sum game in the short-term.'

A potential counterweight to any shifting effect seen through governmental responses to SARS is spill-over benefits that increased SARS vigilance might produce for infectious disease surveillance and response. Efforts to make surveillance systems more prepared for the emergence of SARS may create positive externalities by generating public health capabilities useful for surveillance and response activities with respect to other infectious diseases. Experts have identified similar synergies between preparedness for bioterrorism and for naturally occurring infectious diseases. WHO's David Heymann (2003a, p. 54) argued, for example, that 'strengthening public health for naturally occurring infectious diseases will ensure detection and response to those that may be deliberately caused.' How much SARS-specific activities produce synergistic spill-over for infectious disease control generally remains to be seen.

Some skeptics have expressed concern about the potential for governments to focus too much on SARS. *Médecins Sans Frontières* (2003b) criticized, for example, the G-8 Action Plan on Health issued in June 2003 because '[t]he only section of the Action Plan that shows determination is for SARS. Diseases that primarily affect poor people and occur in places of little consequence to the global economy are not treated with the same urgency.' If responses to SARS create public health systems only tuned to severe epidemic diseases with high cross-border mobility, then post-Westphalian governance might risk becoming as irrelevant in the future as the IHR became for today's infectious disease problems.

Ironically, the best way for public health to break the sustainability conundrum is to hope for repeated crises that keep the need for robust public health constantly at the top of the political agenda nationally and internationally. In the last decade, crises have kept coming in the form of emerging and re-emerging infectious diseases, the appalling growth of the HIV/AIDS pandemic, the global problem of antimicrobial resistance, the threat of bioterrorism, and the emergence of SARS. Even with this parade of pathogenic horribles, the sustainability of post-Westphalian governance remains in doubt. Because of the sustainability conundrum, a seasonal struggle with SARS might paradoxically be the best thing for the sustainability of post-Westphalian public health governance.

Crossing with baggage: Public health's Westphalian core

A central theme of post-Westphalian public health is the disciplining of sovereignty in ways that contribute to global health governance and the production of global public goods for health. The disciplining of sovereignty witnessed in the governance strategies utilized in the SARS outbreak might, if not tempered, obscure recognition that public health as an activity retains a Westphalian core. Public health's Westphalian core restrains the potential of post-Westphalian governance. Public health crossed its post-Westphalian Rubicon with baggage from the Westphalian era.

Theoretically and practically, state-centrism marks public health as a discipline and activity. To the extent it exists, public health theory has focused almost exclusively on the role of governments in protecting population health. Traditionally, experts conceived of public health as a 'public good,' a service or resource that only governments can adequately produce (Institute of Medicine, 1988, p. 7; Gostin, 2000, p. 4). Non-state actors, whether individuals or private enterprises, have neither the incentives nor the resources to supply protection of population health. Public health histories reflect this state-centrism because they reflect the primacy of governmental policy (Rosen, 1958; Porter, 1999). Legal analysis of public health likewise teaches how central the government is to the pursuit of public health (Gostin, 2000, pp. 5–11). The state-centric nature of public health theory and practice does not mean that the government supplies all elements of a public health system, but it underscores that the government's responsibilities for population health are critical, comprehensive, and continuous.

Public health's traditional state-centrism reflects the fact that humanity is divided politically into sovereign states. As a matter of political structure, public health has always been constructed with the boundaries of sovereignty in mind. Westphalian public health developed as public health problems, particularly infectious diseases, generated cross-border frictions among governments. The Westphalian approach was also consistent with public health theory's emphasis on the role of the government in providing for the public's health because this approach was intergovernmental in nature.

Post-Westphalian public health breaks with the state-centrism of public health's past in its emphasis on global health governance and the production of global public goods for health. The state no longer retains a monopoly on the protection of the public's health within its territory. The SARS outbreak illustrated the importance of global surveillance, coordinated by WHO, to state responses to the threat. No state could respond effectively to SARS without accessing the mechanisms of global health governance and contributing to the production of global public goods for health. China tried and failed miserably in acting as if the Chinese government retained a monopoly on public health governance within China.

The involvement of non-state actors in epidemiological surveillance and the empowerment of WHO to use that involvement in global infectious disease responses change the context in which states exercise their public health sovereignty. At the same time, public health retains a Westphalian core because the state's responsibilities for the public's health remain critical, comprehensive, and continuous in this new governance environment.

Post-Westphalian public health governance will not work unless states create and maintain strong national public health systems. Global health governance changes the context in which states exercise their sovereignty, but effective public health responses still require sovereignty to be exercised effectively. Global health governance, and the production of global public goods for health, remain dependent on the quality of national public health governance. Non-state actors may have provided epidemiological information on SARS to WHO, but only state actors could take the actions necessary to contain the outbreak. The Westphalian core of public health appears each time WHO or public health experts stress the importance of national public health capabilities to successful global management of infectious diseases.

In the Westphalian template, state-centrism was largely a matter of jurisdiction because the principles of sovereignty, non-intervention, and consent-based international law created boundaries demarcating the limits of political and legal power. Under this construct, a state's decision whether to report disease events in its territory rested entirely with the state. The state could agree to report certain disease events through international law, but intergovernmental organizations were severely limited in their ability to use non-governmental information about disease events in that jurisdiction.

In the post-Westphalian context, state-centrism in public health is not largely a matter of jurisdiction because the development of global health governance has eroded the significance of formal jurisdictional boundaries. For example, the global flow of non-governmental epidemiological information drastically alters a state's decision whether to report disease outbreaks in its jurisdiction. The state has lost effective 'jurisdiction' over both epidemiological information related to its territory and the decision whether to report disease events. State-centrism in post-Westphalian public health is more a matter of capabilities than jurisdiction. In other words, does the state possess the requisite capabilities to deal with infectious disease threats in a world characterized by globalized anarchy?

A state-centrism of capabilities represents an enormous challenge for post-Westphalian public health governance for two basic reasons. First, post-Westphalian governance possesses no 'power of the purse' because decisions on whether and how to use public resources for population health remain the exclusive domain of sovereign states. Second, a state-centrism of capabilities focuses attention on the massive gaps that exist in public health capacity between the developed and developing worlds. These gaps create the need for resource redistribution from rich to poor if public health capabilities globally are to be improved.

This conclusion resonates with arguments made by, for example, WHO's Commission on Macroeconomics and Health (2001) for significant increases in spending by industrialized countries to help developing countries address infectious disease and other public health problems. This analysis also echoes the resource redistribution scheme at the heart of the Global Fund to Fight AIDS, Tuberculosis, and Malaria. Other global public–private partnerships for health involve resource expenditures to facilitate improvements in health in the developing world, such as occurs with the ventures to develop new drugs for malaria and tuberculosis.

The need for large-scale resource redistribution to advance post-Westphalian public health creates a political dynamic reminiscent of the Westphalian world – the strong have disproportionate influence over governance dynamics. Appeals to the great powers to fund global public health improvements are everywhere in the relevant literature. For example, Heymann (2003a, p. 54) argues that '[i]t is in the interest of industrialized countries to provide the resources and partnership necessary for strengthening public health systems in developing countries if international public health security from naturally occurring and deliberately caused infectious diseases is to be achieved.' The next section of this chapter explores the role of the great powers in post-Westphalian public health in more detail, but it is important to note now that the disproportionate influence of powerful countries in the dynamic created by a state-centrism of capabilities forms part of the Westphalian core of public health that continues to affect public health governance efforts.

In addition to the problem of resources, a state-centrism of capabilities is difficult to manage because its management requires 'beyond the border' reforms that penetrate deeply into a state's sovereignty. Chapter 3 described the shift in international public health policy on infectious disease control from horizontal to vertical approaches in order to communicate the need for international health governance to get inside states to reduce infectious disease prevalence at the source. A state-centrism of capabilities likewise creates the need for global health governance to seek reforms in national public health policies that go well beyond traditional at-the-border strategies embedded, for example, in the IHR.

'Beyond the border' public health reforms are difficult to craft and implement successfully for two reasons. First, experts recognize that the processes of globalization erode a state's capabilities to control activities and events in its territory. Scholte (2000, p. 46) refers to this phenomenon as 'deterritorialization,' a term that also captures the end of a state-centrism based on jurisdiction. This phenomenon of deterritorialization stands behind the frequent arguments in public health literature that infectious disease problems will only be effectively addressed through increased international cooperation because no state can control pathogenic microbes on its own.

The erosion effect of globalization on sovereignty is worse for developing countries because (1) they are less well-equipped economically and politically to manage the rigors of globalized markets, trade, and commerce; and (2) they bear a higher burden of morbidity and mortality from infectious diseases, which acts as a drag on the economic development of these societies. In short, much of the world's population lives in countries ill-equipped to manage pathogenic threats of any kind, globalized or localized. Help from outside is required.

Global health governance faces the challenge of enhancing the public health capabilities of the weaker members of the international society. This challenge is difficult because sovereignty continues to rear its head and complicate the global management of a state-centrism of capabilities. The HIV/AIDS pandemic illustrates the continuing problems sovereignty poses in post-Westphalian public health. Andrew Price-Smith (2002, p. 136) observed the following:

> ...[S]overeignty has in fact had important negative ramifications for the continuing proliferation of the global infectious disease threat, particularly since concerned state and non-state actors may not intervene in seriously affected countries without that country's explicit permission to do so. In the case of states such as South Africa and Zimbabwe, where there remains an enduring culture of denial regarding HIV/AIDS, this means that the international community has little choice but to stand by and watch the ruling elites of these countries preside over the destruction of their populaces.

Public health's lingering Westphalian core produces, thus, the need for not only massive resource redistribution from rich to poor but also management of sovereignty on the part of both giving and receiving states. The state-centrism of capabilities creates dissonance between sovereign states, recalling how donor–recipient relations in the post-World War II period were a political and ideological battleground in international health (Loughlin and Berridge, 2002, p. 16). Wealthy states will not exercise their sovereignty over their financial resources in a manner equivalent to writing blank checks for low-income countries to spend as they see fit. Recipient countries, on the other hand, will bristle if donor governments place too many demands on how the recipient countries use international assistance. The likely outcome of this dynamic is limited, highly-conditioned assistance that does not adequately support global management of infectious disease threats. On the other side of the Rubicon, post-Westphalian public health confronts a potential quagmire linked to the continuing impact of sovereignty.

Realpolitik over the Rubicon: Post-Westphalian public health and the great powers

As Chapter 3 analyzed, Westphalian public health bore the imprint of the great powers of the international system. The humbling of a rising great power, China, by global health governance mechanisms in the SARS outbreak provides evidence that the great powers' influence in post-Westphalian public health is diminished. The great powers did not control or manipulate key aspects of the global campaign against SARS, including the use of non-governmental surveillance information against China and WHO's use of global alerts and travel warnings. Even the world's hegemon, the United States, supported (after some grumbling) the resolutions in the World Health Assembly that solidified the strategies utilized in the SARS outbreak. The SARS outbreak witnessed the great powers as humble members of the global village rather than its haughty overlords.

While the shift from Westphalian to post-Westphalian public health signals a change in the role of the great powers in public health governance, some caution is in order with respect to this role. Post-Westphalian public health is not devoid of politics or immune to the effects of power. In some respects, the context of post-Westphalian public health heightens the importance of the great powers in new ways. To begin, the resources needed to address the capabilities gap discussed in the previous section have to come from the more affluent nations of the world, which are, by and large, the political and economic great powers of the international system – the United States, European Union, and Japan.

Great-power influence in the Westphalian era was not manifested in schemes of resource redistribution for public health; rather, this influence manifested itself in the nature of the governance regime built to mitigate the burden infectious diseases posed to the commerce and populations of powerful nations. As the handling of the SARS outbreak demonstrates, the Westphalian regime built by the great powers has collapsed. Yet, the international community faces no other option but to turn again to the great powers to take the lead in shaping post-Westphalian public health because of the desperate need for material resources to improve global infectious disease control capabilities.

The inescapable need for great-power involvement and leadership explains the tone of much of the literature on emerging and re-emerging infectious diseases in the 1990s and early 2000s, which attempted to frame the growing microbial threat in terms of the self-interests of the great powers, particularly the United States. The titles and sub-titles of some leading reports send a clear message: *America's Vital Interest in Global Health* (Institute of Medicine, 1997); *The Global Infectious Disease Threat and Its Implications for the United States* (National Intelligence Council, 2000); *Why Health is Important to U.S. Foreign Policy* (Kassalow, 2001); *Health, Security, and U.S. Global Leadership* (Ban, 2001); *Reconciling U.S. National Security and Public Health Policy* (Brower and Chalk, 2003).

These, and other, attempts to re-engage the world's hegemon with global public health appeal to the self-interests of the United States. *America's Vital Interest in Global Health* lists three strategic rationales for US engagement: 'protecting our people,' 'enhancing our economy,' and 'advancing our international interests' (Institute of Medicine, 1997). *Why Health is Important to U.S. Foreign Policy* provides a classic example of this appeal when it argues that the United States should make health a foreign policy concern out of 'narrow self-interest' and 'enlightened self-interest' (Kassalow, 2001). William Foege (2003) links US interests to global health by focusing on the US military and protecting US citizens, and stressing that 'healthy societies provide better markets for US goods and healthy societies are able to provide less expensive goods for sale to the United States.' More conceptually, economic approaches to global public health problems, advanced by the World Bank (1993) and the Commission on Macroeconomics and Health (2001) attempt to provide the great powers of the international system with direct, selfish motivations to engage more intensively in international health activities.

Arguments that tie progress in global public health to the self-interests of the United States are nothing new. In 1971, for example, Representative Hugh L. Carey, arguing in favor of the proposed International Health Agency Act of 1971, said the following:

> Again as a practical matter it is in our self-interest to find and fight disease in foreign lands as a safeguard for our own population. Pandemic diseases respect no borders... A second practical consideration is that improved health among the developing peoples abroad means more viable young nations and better hopes for a peaceful environment throughout the world. I submit that health care is our lowest cost form of international security and protection against war and violence... Third, improved health overseas in all age brackets means expanding consumer markets and increased trade for US products. (International Health Agency Act Hearings, 1971, p. 5)

The emphasis on the health vulnerability, economic costs and opportunities, security concerns, and foreign-policy objectives of the great powers present in much of the literature on emerging and re-emerging infectious diseases in the 1990s and early 2000s has a Westphalian ring to it. The pattern that emerges from these contemporary efforts to re-engage the great powers in global public health could be taken from the pages of nineteenth-century international health diplomacy. We see again emphasis on economic, military, and geopolitical aspects of infectious disease threats from the perspective of the great powers.

These observations are not meant to criticize those who have been appealing to the self-interests of the United States and other powerful countries to show leadership on global public health problems. These appeals reflect not only the consequences of the state-centrism of capabilities (discussed above) but also the continuation of a special role for the great powers in post-Westphalian public health. Ilona Kickbusch's

(2003, p. 199) question for global health governance – 'What role for the realist American hegemony?' – is significant in the post-Westphalian world because US 'hegemonic power defines the strategies proposed in the global forum' (Kickbusch, 2002, p. 139). This great power role is different from the functions the great powers served in the Westphalian period but nonetheless places these countries in a very influential position vis-à-vis the global management of infectious diseases.

Success in elevating global infectious disease threats on foreign policy agendas of the great powers in the post-Westphalian period may have the ironic effect of rejuvenating Westphalian patterns of behavior. If powerful countries increase and sustain their national interests in connection with infectious diseases, then they might take firmer control of infectious disease diplomacy. Evidence for this dynamic is already apparent in the context of HIV/AIDS.

The United States' Emergency Plan for AIDS Relief (Emergency Plan), announced by President Bush in January 2003, now overshadows one of the highest profile experiments in global health governance, the Global Fund to Fight AIDS, Tuberculosis, and Malaria (Global Fund). The United States unilaterally controls how the vast majority of the Emergency Plan's $15 billion will be spent, with only a small amount being channeled – with conditions attached – into the Global Fund. Supporters of the Global Fund have criticized the Emergency Plan's unilateralism (Fidler, 2003c, p. 141). The Emergency Plan represents a significantly higher political and financial commitment by the United States to the global HIV/AIDS problem, but the US approach in the Emergency Plan perhaps shares more characteristics with Westphalian than post-Westphalian public health because the United States is using its material power to set and dominate the agenda.

The role of the great powers in post-Westphalian governance may also evolve in ways that create dissonance as opposed to harmony in the world politics of public health. Technological innovations and the harnessing of these by international organizations and non-state actors have broken the traditional 'great power concert' that dominated infectious disease diplomacy in the Westphalian period. This great power concert created a governance structure for infectious diseases that catered mainly to the public health and trade interests of the great powers. The concert created institutions primarily to facilitate protection of these interests and secondarily to provide technical and financial assistance to less powerful nations.

A new kind of 'great power concert' may come to dominate post-Westphalian public health governance. This concert may abandon its traditional ambivalence and indifference toward public health in other parts of the world and act in more determined ways to address the globalized nature of pathogenic threats, which will include improving public health capabilities in the developing world. The great powers may take on something akin to a stewardship or trusteeship role concerning global public health, using their material resources to dictate the content and pace of reform within developing countries. Kurt Campbell and Philip Zelikow (2003, p. 6) have argued, for example, that it 'might be beneficial to consider new international institutions... to take on burdens of field intervention or even "trusteeship."' Vertical public health strategies will then have a political edge not present in the Westphalian context because they will challenge (if not brush aside) developing-country appeals to sovereignty and non-intervention. Done in a heavy-handed way, a stewardship or trustee role on the part of the great powers will take on an imperial quality that will undermine its long-term chances of success.

This new kind of 'great power concert' has better prospects of succeeding if it channels and disciplines its supremacy in power through principles designed to address globalized disease threats. The SARS outbreak illustrates the importance of some of these principles, including: (1) expanding epidemiological surveillance to include non-governmental sources of information; (2) supporting the free and open flow of epidemiological information nationally and globally; (3) strengthening and empowering WHO in terms of both its surveillance and response capabilities; and (4) creating sustainable frameworks through which national surveillance and response capabilities can be enhanced in the developing world. The strategic objective for the new 'great power concert' is to integrate horizontal and vertical governance strategies in a comprehensive, interdependent manner.

The handling of the SARS outbreak provides evidence of the potential for the new 'great power concert' to achieve the strategic objective of integrated global health governance. The expansion of epidemiological surveillance to include non-governmental information helped the global campaign against SARS, as illustrated by the World Health Assembly's confirmation of this approach at its May 2003 meeting. WHO's battle with China over the flow of epidemiological information underscores the critical importance of governments allowing the free and open flow of disease outbreak information. WHO member states recognized the importance of empowering and strengthening WHO in light of WHO's revolutionary actions during the SARS outbreak. Finally, the SARS outbreak revealed the gaping need for public health capabilities to be improved in every nation, especially developing countries.

Importantly, the great powers of the international system seem committed to the first three of the principles described above, including the exercise of autonomous power by WHO in circumstances such as those that arose in the SARS outbreak. An integrated strategy will not, however, coalesce without the great powers' commitment to leading the creation of sustainable frameworks for national public health reforms in the developing world. Whether that commitment takes shape in the wake of SARS still remains to be seen.

Reflecting on prospects for world order, Hedley Bull (1977, p. 315) argued that 'a consensus, founded upon the great powers alone, that does not take into account the demands of those Asian, African and Latin American countries that are weak and poor . . . who represent a majority of states and of the world's population, cannot be expected to endure.' This insight can be reformulated for thinking about the prospects of post-Westphalian public health.

A 'great power concert' for global public health requires a consensus among the great powers that takes seriously the threat of globalized pathogens – a consensus the SARS outbreak has done much to stimulate and solidify. But any governance strategies built on this consensus cannot be expected to endure if the public health travails of the majority of states and of the world's population are not taken into account and mitigated. As Kickbusch (2003, p. 200) warned, '[i]ncreasingly the developing world is watching with scepticism how "global priorities" become just another linguistic expression of the interest of rich and powerful countries, and the plight of the poor is not improved, despite increasing globalist rhetoric.'

Building a great power concert sensitive to the health needs of the developing world is difficult because, as Helen Epstein (2003, p. 15) writes, '[t]he reason the health crisis in developing countries is so serious is precisely because it is possible for rich nations to prosper even with billions of sick and hungry people in the world.' In the post-Westphalian world of public health, the great powers are confronted with a challenge and responsibility that, historically, has proved beyond their capabilities.

Germs don't recognize Rubicons: Confronting the axis of illness

Although post-Westphalian governance mechanisms helped stop SARS dead in its tracks in 2003, those involved in the global campaign against this new threat understand all too well that the potential for microbial trouble has not abated because of the SARS success. Post-Westphalian public health is vulnerable to an 'axis of illness.' The axis of illness represents linkages between five interdependent elements that act together to stimulate microbial emergence and spread. The axis presents challenges to post-Westphalian public health governance that reveal weaknesses in such governance, weaknesses that may call for governance approaches even more radical than those solidified and ushered in by the SARS outbreak.

The axis of illness represents a way to capture why infectious diseases pose such a global public health threat today and to illustrate how difficult post-Westphalian governance for infectious diseases will be. This concept builds on analyses that focus on the various factors that are involved in the emergence and spread of infectious diseases. For example, the seminal 1992 report from the Institute of Medicine (1992, p. 47) listed six factors in disease emergence: human demographics and behavior; technology and industry; economic development and land use; international travel and commerce; microbial adaptation and change; and breakdown of public health measures. Identifying such factors helps communicate the message that infectious disease emergence and re-emergence is an interdependent relationship between the microbe, host, and the environment in which they interact (see Figure 8.1).

The most recent Institute of Medicine report on microbial threats (2003, p. 60) expands the factors in infectious disease emergence from six to 13, which emphasizes the enormous complexity of the phenomenon of disease emergence and spread (see Table 8.1).

The Institute of Medicine's 2003 report sees infectious disease emergence arising from the convergence of genetic and biological factors; physical environmental factors; ecological factors; and social, political, and economic factors. The convergence of these interlocking factors

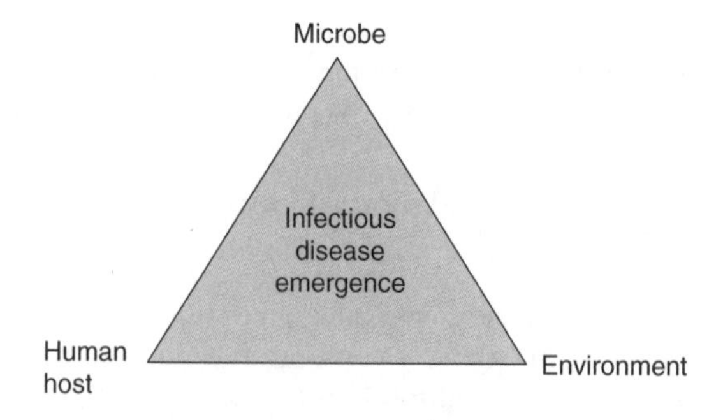

Figure 8.1 Host–microbe–environment interdependence

Table 8.1 Institute of Medicine (2003) factors in infectious disease emergence

• Microbial adaptation and change	• International trade and travel
• Human susceptibility to infection	• Technology and industry
• Climate and weather	• Breakdown of public health systems
• Changing ecosystems	• Poverty and social inequality
• Human demographics and behavior	• War and famine
• Economic development and land use	• Lack of political will
	• Intent to harm

determines the nature of the interaction between the human and the microbe.

Similary, the 'axis of illness' idea provides a way to organize factors of infectious disease emergence to simplify this complex phenomenon by assigning the factors to five overarching categories (see Table 8.2).

The category of 'microbial resilience' captures the importance of microbial, genetic, and biological factors that power pathogenic evolution and its relationship to the human body. 'Human mobility' emphasizes the role played by international trade, travel, and migration in disease emergence, including the contributions technology has made in increasing the speed, scope, and impact of human mobility. The category of 'social determinants of health' focuses attention on the underlying societal problems that foster microbial penetration of populations. Social determinants of health are under constant pressure from the other

Table 8.2 Factors of emergence in five categories

Category	*Factors from Institute of Medicine (2003)*
Microbial resilience	Microbial adaptation and change; human susceptibility to infection
Human mobility	International trade and travel; human demographics and behavior; technology and industry
Social determinants of health	Poverty and social inequalities; war and famine; climate and weather; human demographics and behavior
Globalization	Economic development and land use; technology and industry; changing ecosystems; human demographics and behavior
Collective action problems	Lack of political will; intent to harm; breakdown of public health measures; poverty and social inequalities; war and famine

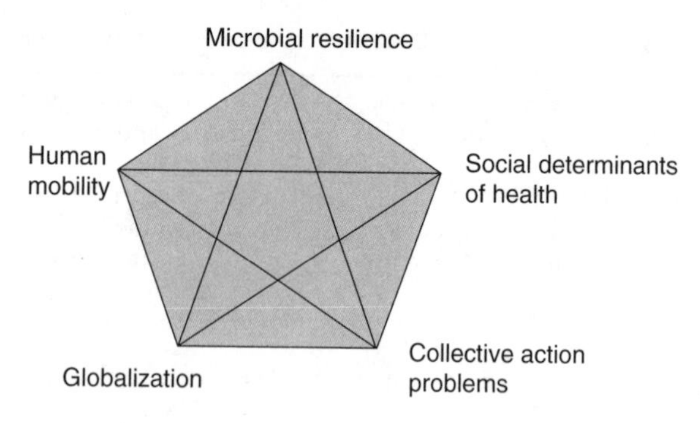

Figure 8.2 The axis of illness

categories in the axis of illness and are undermined by factors, such as the breakdown in public health measures, that weaken the effort. 'Globalization' refers to factors that accelerate economic development, technology, industry, and culture in ways that deterritorialize human behavior. The category of 'collective action problems' refers to the governance challenges created by infectious disease emergence at national, international, and global levels.

The axis of illness forms as these five categories interact to foster the emergence and spread of infectious diseases (see Figure 8.2). It is important to stress that each category connects with the others directly and indirectly in a dynamic process. For example, the processes of globalization directly affect human mobility by making faster transportation technologies available. Globalization affects collective action problems directly and indirectly through exacerbating problems with social determinants of health and accelerating human mobility. Of most relevance for my purposes is how the axis of illness highlights the daunting governance challenges the emergence and re-emergence of infectious diseases present. Successful management of the collective action problems is only the beginning, because those solutions have to bear, in some sustainable fashion, the force produced by the interdependence of microbial resilience, human mobility, social determinants of health, and globalization.

The SARS outbreak underscores each element of the axis of illness and the challenges it poses for states, international organizations, and non-state actors. The emergence of a virus never before seen in animals or humans demonstrates that microbial resilience played a role in this outbreak. SARS-CoV took advantage of opportunities human behavior presented and forced the world of public health and science to ponder the mysteries of yet another new, dangerous virus. The speed with which SARS-CoV apparently jumped from animals to human and then triggered a local, regional, and global epidemic is evidence of the potent miasma the global village creates for the microbial world.

SARS reinforces the effectiveness of human mobility, in combination with the processes of globalization, as a means of spreading pathogenic microbes. WHO's resort to historically unprecedented travel advisories against specific geographic areas illustrates how dangerous global travel can be in the context of infectious diseases. The economic damage caused to SARS-affected countries from lost tourism and business-related travel is a further indication of how dependent the globalized world is on air travel. The emergence of post-Westphalian public health governance does nothing to lessen this dependence. This element of the axis of illness will only continue to grow in importance.

The SARS outbreak also illustrated the importance of social determinants of health in disease emergence. The role likely played by the sale of exotic animals for food or medicine in southern China represents a socially determined risk to health, perhaps exacerbated by China's mid-August 2003 decision to lift the ban on the sale and consumption of exotic animals it imposed during the SARS outbreak (National Intelligence Council, 2003, p. 9). Commentators noted the role poverty, unemployment, migrant labor practices, and lack of access to medical services played in China's SARS outbreak (Huang, 2003, pp. 70–1; National Intelligence Council, 2003, p. 9). Experts also observed that SARS' appearance in a number of relatively affluent nations with modern public health and health care systems significantly helped the global campaign bring SARS under control. Fears that SARS may gain a foothold in poor countries and regions with substantial sick and malnourished populations, such as sub-Saharan Africa (National Intelligence Council, 2003, p. 24), further highlight social determinants of health as factors in infectious disease emergence and spread.

The SARS outbreak also reflects the role collective action problems can play in disease emergence. At the national level, the epidemic revealed weaknesses and problems in the public health capabilities of many countries affected by the epidemic. As noted earlier, many of the seriously SARS-affected countries, such as Canada, Singapore, Hong Kong, and Taiwan, were nations with relatively sophisticated public health and health care systems, and SARS stretched these systems to breaking point. The SARS outbreak also exposed serious deficiencies in China's public health and health care capabilities. Experts even questioned the public health preparedness of nations not seriously affected by the outbreak, such as the United States. Although the SARS epidemic did not heavily affect developing countries, particularly those in Africa, fear remained high during the outbreak that SARS would invade nations with the least capability to respond to such a disease threat. All these examples prove that national collective action problems concerning public health constitute a robust link in the axis of illness.

The move toward global health governance, especially the incorporation of non-governmental information in global surveillance, is an explicit indication that intergovernmentalism as a collective action response had proved inadequate for infectious disease control purposes. Similarly, WHO's radical actions during the SARS outbreak – in publicly confronting China's duplicity and lies and in issuing geographically-specific travel advisories – were actions not supported at the time taken by the existing intergovernmental and international legal regimes in place on infectious disease control.

SARS also illustrates the role globalization plays in disease emergence. International political economists have analyzed the growing loss of the state's control over its domestic economy caused by global economic interdependence and integration (Strange, 1995, pp. 160–1). The globalization of markets 'has intensified economic competition and increased pressure on governments to reduce expenditures, including the funding of public health programs, leaving states increasingly unprepared to deal with emerging disease problems' (Fidler, 1996, p. 78). Globalization feeds into the creation and perpetuation of public health vulnerabilities. Similarly, the loss of economic control complicates the state's ability to address socio-economic problems, such as poverty and urbanization, or to slow down environmental degradation resulting from economic activity. The globalization of markets for goods, capital, and services exacerbates social, economic, and environmental problems, particularly in the developing world, that provide opportunities for pathogenic microbes.

This element of the axis of illness can be seen clearly in the SARS problem in China. The move to a more market-based economy, increasingly integrated with the rest of the world, resulted in declining government funding and commitment to China's public health and health care systems. Globalization's weakening of China's ability to deal with infectious diseases is reflected not only in the SARS outbreak but also the growing HIV/AIDS problem in that country.

Post-Westphalian public health governance has given states, international organizations, and non-state actors new strategies and mechanisms for reacting to disease emergence and re-emergence. These new governance strategies create potential for better global surveillance and response activities. Global health governance and the production of global public goods for health target one element of the axis of illness – the collective action problems. Less clear is whether post-Westphalian public health contains new strategies for preventing the emergence and spread of infectious diseases. Prevention strategies would include addressing the social determinants of health by mitigating the deeply-rooted social, economic, and environmental problems that nurture microbial emergence and spread.

Given the gaps in public health capabilities and economic resources, prevention strategies might involve more significant interventions into the domestic affairs of sovereign states that even post-Westphalian public health governance, at its present stage, does not contemplate. While proposals for improving response capabilities (e.g., surveillance and intervention) have been made, there has been little, or no, discussion of 'pre-emptive' public health governance in the aftermath of SARS. In addition to the long list of infectious diseases that have emerged or re-emerged in the last three decades, SARS may suggest that the forces of globalization mean that post-Westphalian public health governance can merely be reactive rather than preventive in resolving the collective action problems that exist.

In this respect, post-Westphalian governance would parallel Westphalian public health – an unwelcome parallel given how events eventually bypassed the Westphalian template in favor of reactive strategies better suited to the exigencies of a globalized world. The axis of illness demonstrates that the germs will continue advancing, placing sustained pressure on post-Westphalian governance. The public health victory achieved in SARS represents only one battle in the confrontation with the axis of illness. The SARS outbreak confirms that conditions on the other side of the post-Westphalian Rubicon still favor the axis.

Mike Ryan is correct – after SARS, there is no going back to the ways of Westphalian public health. Public health's 'new world order' remains, however, a work very much in progress. This chapter analyzed vulnerabilities that post-Westphalian public health governance might face in the coming years. That vulnerabilities exist is hardly a surprise or cause for panic. In addition, having witnessed the astonishing achievement of SARS containment, most people dedicated to public health would much rather confront these vulnerabilities and the challenges, known and unknown, that lie ahead with the arsenal of post-Westphalian governance than without it.

9
Conclusion: Governing Infectious Diseases in Globalized Anarchy

The tipping point

The argument in this book that SARS is the first post-Westphalian pathogen provided the foundation for exploring how the SARS outbreak reflected the emergence and use of new forms of governance for the global threat of infectious diseases. This exploration produced a political pathology of the SARS outbreak that revealed governance of infectious disease threats completing a transition from Westphalian to post-Westphalian strategies. The SARS outbreak did not initiate this transition or create all the strategies implemented to contain this new disease because the move from Westphalian public health governance was underway prior to SARS.

As Ilona Kickbusch (2003, p. 200) observed before the SARS outbreak, '[w]e are in transition from what seemed a relatively reliable, state defined and structured world of international health to a diffuse political space of global health in which new forms of distributed power and new patterns of power-sharing emerge.' The political pathology of SARS constructed in this book demonstrates, however, that the SARS outbreak represents a historic moment in public health governance because it marks the point at which a new governance paradigm for global infectious disease threats truly came of age.

I have emphasized in this book the extent to which the handling of the SARS outbreak demonstrates the governance revolution that has taken place with respect to infectious diseases. The global campaign against SARS bears no resemblance to Westphalian public health governance. The Westphalian tenets of sovereignty, non-intervention, and the disciplining of sovereignty through consent-based international law did not determine the behavior of states, WHO, and non-state actors in the global struggle against the spread of SARS. The great powers did not dictate events during the SARS outbreak as they had done during the heyday of Westphalian public health. Instead, the political pathology of SARS reveals global health governance and the production of global public goods for health as new and promising features of a post-Westphalian form of infectious disease governance.

The 'global health governance' and 'global public goods for health' concepts were alive in public health discourse and practice prior to the SARS outbreak, but the management of this outbreak brought the concepts to impressive life in ways their previous uses had not achieved. Although glimpses of the potential of these concepts occurred prior to SARS, particularly in the development of the Global Outbreak Alert and Response Network (Global Network) and various public–private partnerships for health, the SARS epidemic constitutes a 'tipping point' for these new governance strategies because they were implemented effectively in the fires of a global public health crisis.

In his well-known book, *The Tipping Point,* Malcom Gladwell (2000) notes that he took the idea of the 'tipping point' from epidemiology, which identifies sharp increases or decreases in the curves of epidemics as tipping points. Gladwell (2000, p. 9) argued that the tipping point is 'that one dramatic moment in an epidemic when everything can change all at once.' These dramatic changes often occur because 'little causes can have big effects' (Gladwell, 2000, p. 9). Such little causes with big effects are linked to something contagious.

In the SARS outbreak, the epidemiological tipping point occurred during Dr Liu Jianlun's stay at the Metropole Hotel in Hong Kong because Dr Liu passed the contagious SARS virus to fellow travelers, who dispersed the syndrome around the world. This small event – an elderly man infected with a virus attending a wedding – triggered a global public health crisis.

The governance tipping point in the epidemic came on 15 March when WHO issued its emergency travel advisory and declared SARS a world-wide health threat. WHO had previously issued a global alert on 12 March because it saw a pattern emerging that required placing the international community on notice; but events immediately following the 12 March alert – reports from Canada about cases of atypical pneumonia on 14 March and the 15 March isolation of the symptomatic Singaporean doctor in Frankfurt en route to Singapore – pushed WHO to a much higher level of concern, which led to the extraordinary events played out in the global campaign to control SARS.

The SARS epidemic can also be considered a more general governance tipping point for global infectious disease control. Although strategies for infectious disease control had already begun to move away from the Westphalian model, the handling of the SARS outbreak has taken this transition to a new level of importance and potential effectiveness that makes any return to Westphalian modes of surveillance unthinkable. As WHO has stressed time and time again, early warning and rapid intervention are critical to the success of managing outbreaks of infectious diseases, particularly new diseases the epidemiology of which is not well understood. Before SARS, WHO had been demonstrating the potential of the Global Network with respect to other outbreaks; but the SARS crisis has taken this approach to another level of significance. Continued refinement, strengthening, and expansion of global health governance on infectious disease surveillance are the tasks now before WHO, states, and non-state actors. The proposed public–private partnership to improve SARS surveillance and response at national levels also confirms the shift toward post-Westphalian strategies on infectious disease control.

Similarly, the successful management of the SARS outbreak depended on the production of global public goods for health, in the form of global surveillance data, best practices for clinicians, and basic scientific information on the coronavirus behind the disease. All these types of information were produced and consumed by global constituencies that included governments, international organizations, non-governmental actors, and concerned individuals around the world. The production, dissemination, and consumption of all these forms of global information were unprecedented. The SARS outbreak gives, thus, the concept of global public goods for health added significance and momentum as post-Westphalian governance for infectious disease control takes shape.

The SARS epidemic also represents a governance tipping point for WHO. The mounting global public health threats, including emerging and re-emerging infectious diseases, identified in the 1990s led to intense scrutiny and criticism of WHO as the leader of international health efforts. The appointment of Gro Harlem Brundtland as Director-General in 1998 was seen by many as important to the rejuvenation of WHO's prestige, influence, and impact. The SARS outbreak has taken WHO's role in public health governance to a point few would have predicted when Brundtland was appointed.

WHO's exercise of independent power during the SARS outbreak in issuing global alerts and geographically-specific travel advisories, and the acquiescence and then formal approval of WHO member states of this authority, represent unprecedented developments in the history of the world politics of public health and perhaps even in the history of international organizations. Outside the context of the European Union, one is hard pressed to think of any other past or present international organization armed with independent authority to take actions that can cause serious economic and political damage to countries.

In addition to these astonishing events, the critical role WHO plays in managing global health governance mechanisms, such as the Global Network, and in the production of global public goods for health, also establishes for the Organization a new level of governance importance international health organizations never possessed in the Westphalian world. No country, not even the United States, could have produced on its own or in conjunction with a few other countries the global response led and coordinated by WHO on SARS. The SARS outbreak highlighted a functional significance for WHO that supersedes the recognition of the need for such an organization present in the Westphalian strategy.

The new way of working

Dr David Heymann, WHO's Executive Director of Communicable Diseases, captured the aftermath of the governance tipping point SARS represents by arguing that '[i]n the 21st century there is a new way of working' (Heymann, 2003b). The political pathology of SARS explored in this book dissects this 'new way of working' in order to show that post-Westphalian public health governance is not an empty academic construct but an approach to global infectious disease threats that is real and that scored an impressive victory during the emergence and spread of the twenty-first century's first new, severe infectious disease threat.

My political pathology of SARS represents only an incomplete, first step in exploring this 'new way of working.' This book hopefully will prove useful in meeting challenges Kickbusch (2003, p. 203) emphasized: 'to identify the key elements of what would constitute a virtuous cycle of health governance and to explore these components with creative and rigorous research.' Further empirical and theoretical research and analysis on the importance of SARS to the task of governing infectious diseases in the post-Westphalian world are in order for many reasons, not least of all to ensure that the pursuit of global health is equipped with analytical tools and information that support the sustainable elevation of public health on the global agendas of states, international organizations, and non-state actors.

While victory in the SARS outbreak of 2002–03 should be savored, all should remember that germs do not recognize victories or defeats. The political pathology of SARS does not predict that post-Westphalian public health governance will exhibit the effectiveness achieved in the SARS outbreak in future attempts at governing infectious diseases. Just as the effectiveness of Westphalian governance cannot be judged by examining only the historic triumph of smallpox eradication, conclusions about the sustainability and effectiveness of post-Westphalian public health cannot be based solely on the successful containment of the initial global outbreak of SARS.

Many experts, including those at WHO, expect SARS to emerge again, perhaps in late 2003 and early 2004. At present, public health experts are not optimistic about the prospects of eradicating SARS (Bell *et al.*, 2003, p. 1191). WHO (2003e-3) has warned that '[t]he reappearance of SARS in the human population would be considered a global public health emergency.' For this reason, national and international public health experts remain on pins and needles concerning the possible return of SARS. In August 2003, concerns were raised that an unusual outbreak of respiratory disease in a nursing home in British Columbia might be SARS (Brown, 2003e). In August 2003, to help ensure that complacency does not return, WHO (2003e-3) issued guidance on the development of a SARS alert mechanism for the post-outbreak period. In addition, WHO (2003f-3) began urging its member states to increase the use of influenza vaccines to help 'reduce cases of respiratory disease that could be mistaken for SARS.'

China still looms large in any future confrontation with SARS, raising concerns about China's attitude should the virus and disease return. As a group of public health experts observed, '[m]any of the solutions to solve the multifaceted puzzle of SARS and to prevent future epidemics must come from China. Without solutions from that country, the degree of difficulty for sustained control of the problem globally is raised still higher' (Breiman *et al.*, 2003, p. 1040). China's clamping down on debate about political reform in the post-SARS period (Pomfret, 2003t) creates worries about whether China will respond transparently and openly if SARS returns. Further, continuing problems with China's policy response to HIV/AIDS (Human Rights Watch, 2003; Pan, 2003) heighten fears that China's political system is not up to the challenge of handling the globalization of disease.

SARS may, thus, have its revenge on global health governance the next time it appears. Beyond SARS, epidemiologists still anticipate the coming of the 'big one' – the next killer pandemic of influenza – for which post-Westphalian public health is definitely not prepared. HIV/AIDS, tuberculosis, and malaria still constitute formidable microbial challenges. Antimicrobial resistance continues to plague infectious disease control. Neglected infectious diseases that predominantly ravage developing countries remain a source of great morbidity and mortality. As the pace and scale of globalization accelerates, the danger of the 'axis of illness' grows exponentially.

These, and other, infectious disease challenges will attack the 'new way of working' as severely as infectious diseases relentlessly assaulted the Westphalian public health. The SARS tipping point means, however, that these and other as yet unanticipated pathogenic crises will be governed through post-Westphalian mechanisms and approaches as opposed to the traditional paradigm of 'international health.' As WHO's Mike Ryan aptly put it, 'there's no going back now.'

The challenge for post-Westphalian public health is to create the conditions necessary for the governance innovations tested in the SARS outbreak to be refined, improved, expanded, and sustained to meet the ongoing threats pathogenic microbes present. The germs will keep coming. The great task for the global community that answered the initial challenge from SARS is to ensure that the 'new way of working' continues to work effectively far into the twenty-first century.

References

Abbassi, K. 1999. 'Changing Sides,' *British Medical Journal*; 318: 865–9.

Allott, P. 1999. 'The Concept of International Law,' *European Journal of International Law*; 10: 31–50.

Annas, G.J. 2002. 'Bioterrorism, Public Health, and Civil Liberties,' *New England Journal of Medicine*; 346: 1337–42.

Arhin-Tenkorang, D. and Conceição, P. 2003. 'Beyond Communicable Disease Control: Health in the Age of Globalization.' In: I. Kaul, P. Conceição, K. Le Goulven, and R.U. Mendoza, eds, *Providing Global Public Goods: Managing Globalization* (Oxford: Oxford University Press, 2003), pp. 484–515.

Ban, J. 2001. *Health, Security, and U.S. Global Leadership* (Washington, D.C.: Chemical and Biological Arms Control Institute).

Bell, D., Jenkins, P., and Hall, J. 2003. 'World Health Organization Global Conference on Severe Acute Respiratory Syndrome,' *Emerging Infectious Diseases*; 9: 1191–2.

Birnie, P.W. and Boyle, A.E. 1992. *International Law and the Environment* (Oxford: Clarendon Press).

Bishop, M.W. 2003. 'Beijing at Its Best – Doing Nothing,' *Taipei Times*, 25 June, at www.taipeitimes.com/News/edit/archive/2003/06/25/2003056693.

Bodansky, D. 1995. 'Customary (and Not So Customary) International Environmental Law,' *Indiana Journal of Global Legal Studies*; 3: 105–19.

Breiman, R.F. *et al.* 2003. 'Role of China in the Quest to Define and Control Severe Acute Respiratory Syndrome,' *Emerging Infectious Diseases*; 9: 1073–41.

Brower, J. and Chalk, P. 2003. *The Global Threat of New and Reemerging Infectious Diseases: Reconciling U.S. National Security and Public Health Policy* (Santa Monica: RAND).

Brown, D.L. 2003a. 'Virus Worry Fades in Toronto, but Concern Lingers; Residents Begin to Pick Up Their Old Routines; Officials Call WHO Travel Advisory Unnecessary,' *Washington Post*, 24 April, at A20.

Brown, D.L. 2003b. 'Canada Disputes SARS Travel Alert; Officials Say Rate of New Cases is Down, but WHO Will Not Rescind Warning,' *Washington Post*, 25 April, at A16.

Brown, D.L. 2003c. 'Canada to Counter SARS Advisory; Toronto is "Safe," Chretien Declares; Marketing Campaign Set,' *Washington Post*, 26 April, at A17.

Brown, D.L. 2003d. 'Canadians Say Guard Lowered Too Quickly; Resurgence of SARS in Toronto Spurs Call for Voluntary Quarantine of 3,400,' *Washington Post*, 28 May, at A15.

Brown, D.L. 2003e. 'WHO Probes SARS-Like Virus in British Columbia,' *Washington Post*, 21 August, at A19.

Brown, D.L. and Connolly, C. 2003. 'WHO Drops Travel Advisory for Toronto,' *Washington Post*, 30 April, at A10.

Brownlie, I. 1998. *Principles of Public International Law*, 5th edn (Oxford: Oxford University Press).

Brundtland, G.H. 2003. *Day One Conclusion: The Response So Far – WHO Global Meeting on SARS*, 17 June, at www.who.int/dg/speeches/2003/kuala_lumpur_ sars/en/.

Bull, H. 1977. *The Anarchical Society: A Study of Order in World Politics* (London: Macmillan).

Buse, K. and Walt, G. 2000a. 'Global Public–Private Partnerships: Part I – A New Development in Health?,' *Bulletin of the World Health Organization*; 78: 549–61.

Buse, K. and Walt, G. 2000b. 'Global Public–Private Partnerships: Part II – What Are the Health Issues for Global Governance?,' *Bulletin of the World Health Organization*; 78: 699–709.

Buse, K. and Walt, G. 2002. 'Globalisation and Multilateral Public–Private Health Partnerships: Issues for Health Policy.' In: K. Lee, K. Buse, and S. Fustukian, eds, *Health Policy in a Globalising World* (Cambridge: Cambridge University Press, 2002), pp. 41–62.

Bush, G.W. 2002. *State of the Union Address*, at www.whitehouse.gov/news/releases/2002/01/20020129-11.html.

Campbell, K.M. and Zelikow, P. 2003. 'Executive Summary.' In: *Biological Security & Public Health: In Search of a Global Treatment*, K.M. Cambell and P. Zelikow, eds (Washington, D.C.: Aspen Institute), pp. 3–6.

Carrns, A., Chase, M., and Naik, G. 2003. 'Mysterious Respiratory Illness Proves Hard to Tally Accurately,' *Wall Street Journal*, 18 March, at D4.

Chang, L. 2003a. 'Spread of SARS Slows in China, Raising Hopes,' *Wall Street Journal*, 13 May, at D8.

Chang, L. 2003b. 'China Wins Praise for SARS Efforts,' *Wall Street Journal*, 14 May, at D4.

Chase, M., Pottinger, M., Mckay, B., and Furhmans, V. 2003. 'Labs Collaborate World-Wide to Identify Deadly Virus,' *Wall Street Journal*, 26 March, at B1.

Chen, K. 2003. 'China is As Good at Fighting SARS as at Hiding It,' *Wall Street Journal*, 4 June, at D3.

Chen, K., Dean, J., and Cherney, E. 2003. 'Is Chinese SARS Dropoff for Real?,' *Wall Street Journal*, 29 May, at D4.

Cherney, E. and L. Chang. 2003. 'Health Officials Fighting SARS are Encouraged by Fewer Cases,' *Wall Street Journal*, 2 June, at B5.

Cohen, M., Fritsch, P., and Pottinger, M. 2003. 'Routine Trip Ends with Deadly Illness,' *Wall Street Journal*, 19 March, at B4K.

Cohen, M., Naik, G., and Pottinger, M. 2003. 'Spreading the Word: Inside the WHO as It Mobilized for War on SARS,' *Wall Street Journal*, 2 May, at A1.

Collin, J. 2003. 'Think Global, Smoke Local: Transnational Tobacco Companies and Cognitive Globalization.' In: K. Lee, ed., *Health Impacts of Globalization: Towards Global Governance* (Basingstoke: Palgrave Macmillan, 2003), pp. 61–85.

Commission on Macroeconomics and Health. 2001. *Macroeconomic and Health: Investing in Health for Economic Development* (Geneva: WHO).

Connolly, C. 2003. 'Outbreak Could Flare This Winter, Experts Say,' *Washington Post*, 22 May, at A02.

Declaration of Alma Ata. 1978. In: *Report of the International Conference on Primary Health Care* (Geneva: WHO).

Declaration on Principles of International Law Concerning Friendly Relations and Cooperation Among States. 1970. In: I. Brownlie, ed., *Basic Documents in International Law*, 4th edn (Oxford: Oxford University Press, 1995), pp. 36–45.

Delon, P.J. 1975. *The International Health Regulations: A Practical Guide* (Geneva: WHO).

Dodgson, R., Lee, K., and Drager, N. 2002. *Global Health Governance: A Conceptual Overview* (Discussion Paper No. 1) (London: Centre on Global Change & Health and WHO).

Dorolle, P. 1969. 'Old Plagues in the Jet Age: International Aspects of Present and Future Control of Communicable Diseases,' *Chronicle of the World Health Organization*; 23: 103–11.

Drosten, C. *et al.* 2003. 'Identification of a Novel Coronavirus in Patients with Severe Acute Respiratory Syndrome,' *New England Journal of Medicine*; 348: 1967–76.

Dunne, T. and Schmidt, B.C. 2001. 'Realism.' In: J. Baylis and S. Smith, eds, *The Globalization of World Politics: An Introduction to International Relations*, 2nd edn (Oxford: Oxford University Press, 2001), pp. 141–61.

The Economist. 2002. 'AIDS: The Next Wave,' *The Economist*, 19 October, p. 75.

The Economist. 2003. 'China's Chernobyl?,' *The Economist*, 26 April, pp. 9–10.

Emerging Infections Hearings. 1995. *Hearings Before the U.S. Senate Committee on Labor and Human Resources*, 104th Congress.

Epstein, H. 2003. 'Memorandum to the President: The Global Health Crisis.' In: K.M. Campbell and P. Zelikow, eds, *Biological Security & Public Health: In Search of a Global Treatment* (Washington, D.C.: Aspen Institute, 2003), pp. 9–15.

Farmer, P. 1999. *Infections and Inequalities: The Modern Plagues* (Berkeley: University of California Press).

Feachem, R.G.A. 2003. 'AIDS Hasn't Peaked Yet – And That's Not the Worst of It,' *Washington Post*, 12 January, at B03.

Fidler, D.P. 1996. 'Globalization, Infectious Diseases, and International Law,' *Emerging Infectious Diseases*; 2: 77–83.

Fidler, D.P. 1997a. 'The Globalization of Public Health: Emerging Infectious Diseases and International Relations,' *Indiana Journal of Global Legal Studies*; 5: 11–51.

Fidler, D.P. 1997b. 'The Return of the Fourth Horseman: Emerging Infectious Diseases and International Law,' *Minnesota Law Review*; 81: 771–868.

Fidler, D.P. 1998. '*Microbialpolitik*: Infectious Diseases and International Relations,' *American University International Law Review*; 14: 1–53.

Fidler, D.P. 1999. *International Law and Infectious Diseases* (Oxford: Clarendon Press).

Fidler, D.P. 2000. *International Law and Public Health: Materials on and Analysis of Global Health Jurisprudence* (Ardsley, NY: Transnational Publishers, Inc.).

Fidler, D.P. 2001a. 'Return of "*Microbialpolitik*,"' *Foreign Policy*; Jan./Feb.: 80–1.

Fidler, D.P. 2001b. 'Challenges to Humanity's Health: The Contributions of International Environmental Law to National and Global Public Health,' *Environmental Law Review*; 31: 10048–78.

Fidler, D.P. 2002. *Global Health Governance: Overview of the Role of International Law in Protecting and Promoting Global Public Health* (Discussion Paper No. 3) (London: Centre on Global Change & Health and WHO).

Fidler, D.P. 2003a. 'Emerging Trends in International Law Concerning Global Infectious Disease Control,' *Emerging Infectious Diseases*; 9: 285–90.

Fidler, D.P. 2003b. *SARS and International Law*. American Society of International Law Insight, April, at www.asil.org/insights/insigh101.htm.

Fidler, D.P. 2003c. 'Racism or *Realpolitik*? U.S. Foreign Policy and the HIV/AIDS Catastrophe in Sub-Saharan Africa,' *Journal of Gender, Race & Justice*; 7: 97–146.

Fidler, D.P., Heymann, D., Ostroff, S., and O'Brien, T. 1997. 'Emerging and Reemerging Infectious Diseases: Challenges for International, National, and State Law,' *International Lawyer*; 31: 773–99.

Fluss, S.S. 1997. 'International Public Health Law: An Overview.' In: R. Detels, *et al*. eds, *Oxford Textbook of Public Health*, 3rd edn Vol. 1 (Oxford: Oxford University Press, 1997), pp. 371–90.

Foege, W.H. 2003. 'Memorandum to the President: Global Health and U.S. National Interests.' In: K.M. Campbell and P. Zelikow, eds, *Biological Security & Public Health: In Search of a Global Treatment* (Washington, D.C.: Aspen Institute, 2003), pp. 17–24.

Frank, S. 2003. 'Suddenly, All Smiles,' *Time* (Canadian edition), 12 May, at 2003 WL 11985677.

Frankel, B. 1996. 'Restating the Realist Case.' In: B. Frankel, ed., *Realism: Restatements and Renewal* (London: Frank Cass), pp. ix-xx.

Fritsch, P., Pottinger, M., and Chang, L. 2003. 'Divergent Asian Response Show Difficulties in Dealing with SARS,' *Wall Street Journal*, 7 April, at A1.

Fuhrmans, V. and Naik, G. 2003. 'The WHO Wants Company Money to Battle SARS,' *Wall Street Journal*, 22 May, at D3.

Garrett, L. 1995. *The Coming Plague: Newly Emerging Diseases in a World Out of Balance* (New York: Penguin Books).

Garrett, L. 1996. 'The Return of Infectious Disease,' *Foreign Affairs*; 75(1): 66–79.

Garrett, L. 2003. *Remarks at Panel on China and SARS: The Crisis and Its Effects on Politics and the Economy*, 2 July.

General Agreement on Tariffs and Trade. 1947. In: World Trade Organization, *The Legal Texts: The Results of the Uruguay Round of Multilateral Trade Negotiations* (Cambridge: Cambridge University Press, 1999), pp. 423–92.

Gerberding, J. 2003. 'Faster ... But Fast Enough? Responding to the Epidemic of Severe Acute Respiratory Syndrome,' *New England Journal of Medicine*; 348: 2030–1.

Giesecke, J. 2003. 'International Health Regulations and Epidemic Control.' In: R.D. Smith, R. Beaglhole, D. Woodward, and N. Drager, eds, *Global Public Goods for Health: Health Economic and Public Health Perspectives* (Oxford: Oxford University Press, 2003), pp. 196–211.

Gladwell, M. 2000. *The Tipping Point: How Little Things Can Make a Big Difference* (New York: Little Brown).

Global Fund to Fight AIDS, Tuberculosis, and Malaria. 2003a. *Overview*, at http://www.globalfundatm.org/overview.html.

Global Fund to Fight AIDS, Tuberculosis, and Malaria. 2003b. *NGOs and Civil Society*, at http://www.globalfundatm.org/ngo_civil.html.

Global Fund to Fight AIDS, Tuberculosis, and Malaria. 2003c. *By-Laws of the Global Fund to Fight AIDS, Tuberculosis, and Malaria*, at http://www.globalfundatm.org/publicdoc/bylaws_uk.pdf.

Global Fund to Fight AIDS, Tuberculosis, and Malaria. 2003d. *Principles*, at http://www.globalfundatm.org/principles.html.

Global Fund to Fight AIDS, Tuberculosis, and Malaria. 2003e. *Press Release: Global Fund Awards $866 Million in Grants to Fight AIDS, TB and Malaria; United States Takes Chair of Global Fund Board; Tommy Thompson is Elected*, 31 January.

Godlee, F. 1994a. 'WHO in Crisis,' *British Medical Journal*; 309: 1424–8.
Godlee, F. 1994b. 'WHO in Retreat: Is It Losing Its Influence?,' *British Medical Journal*; 309: 1491–5.
Godlee, F. 1997. 'WHO Reform and Global Health: Radical Restructuring is the Only Way Ahead,' *British Medical Journal*; 314: p. 1359.
Goldgeier, J. 2003. 'Will SARS Be the Chinese Chernobyl?,' *Los Angeles Times*, 23 April, at B13.
Goodman, N.M. 1971. *International Health Organizations and Their Work*, 2nd edn (London: Churchill Livingstone).
Gore, A. 1996. *Address Before the National Council for International Health*, 12 June.
Gostin, L.O. 2000. *Public Health Law: Power, Duty, Restraint* (Berkeley: University of California Press).
Grein, T.W. *et al.* 2000. 'Rumors of Disease in the Global Village: Outbreak Verification,' *Emerging Infectious Diseases*; 6: 97–102.
Grewe, W.G. 2000. *The Epochs of International Law* (M. Byers, trans.) (Berlin: Walter de Gruyter).
Hamburg, M.A. 2003. Testimony of Margaret A. Hamburg, M.D., Vice President of Biological Programs, Nuclear Threat Initiative, U.S. House of Representatives Committee on Government Reform, 9 April.
Harding, C. and Lim, C.L. 1999. 'The Significance of Westphalia: An Archaeology of the International Legal Order.' In: C. Harding and C.L. Lim, eds, *Renegotiating Westphalia: Essays and Commentary on the European and Conceptual Foundations of Modern International Law* (The Hague: M. Nijhoff Publishers, 1999): pp. 1–23.
Health Organization of the League of Nations. 1923. Scheme for the Permanent Health Organization of the League of Nations, 7 July 1923. In: *League of Nations Official Journal* (1923), p. 1050.
Health Organization of the League of Nations. 1931. *Health* (Geneva: Health Organization of the League of Nations).
Heinzl, M. 2003. 'The SARS Outbreak: WHO Will Review Toronto Advisory,' *Wall Street Journal*, 28 April, at A8.
Heinzl, M. and Chipello, C.J. 2003. 'Toronto is Put on Travel Watch, Angering Officials,' *Wall Street Journal*, 24 April, at D5.
Heymann, D.L. 2002. 'The Microbial Threat in Fragile Times: Balance Known and Unknown Risks,' *Bulletin of the World Health Organization*; 80: p. 179.
Heymann, D.L. 2003a. 'Memorandum to the President: Emerging and Epidemic-Prone Diseases: Threats to Public Health Security.' In: K.M. Campbell and P. Zelikow, eds, *Biological Security & Public Health: In Search of a Global Treatment* (Washington, D.C.: Aspen Institute, 2003), pp. 49–55.
Heymann, D.L. 2003b. Testimony of David L. Heymann, Executive Director, Communicable Diseases, World Health Organization, Hearing on Severe Acute Respiratory Syndrome Threat, before the Committee on Health, Education, Labor, and Pensions of the U.S. Senate, 7 April.
Hiatt, F. 2003. 'Lies in the Absence of Liberty,' *Washington Post*, 14 April, at A17.
Hinsley, F.H. 1963. *Power and the Pursuit of Peace: Theory and Practice in the History of Relations Between States* (Cambridge: Cambridge University Press).
Howard-Jones, N. 1950. 'Origins of International Health Work,' *British Medical Journal* (May 6, 1950), 1032–7.

Howard-Jones, N. 1975. *The Scientific Background of the International Sanitary Conferences 1851–1938* (Geneva: WHO).
Huang, Y. 2003. *Mortal Peril: Public Health in China and Its Security Implications* (Health and Security Series Special Report No. 7) (Washington, D.C.: Chemical and Biological Arms Control Institute).
Human Rights Watch. 2003. *Locked Doors: The Human Rights of People Living with HIV/AIDS in China* (Washington, D.C.: Human Rights Watch).
Hunt, P. 2003. *The Right of Everyone to the Enjoyment of the Highest Attainable Standard of Physical and Mental Health: Report of the Special Rapporteur*. UN Doc. E/CN.4/2003/58, 13 February.
Hutzler, C. 2003a. 'WHO Seeks an Investigation of Disease in Beijing,' *Wall Street Journal*, 10 April, at A10.
Hutzler, C. 2003b. 'Chinese Officials Concede SARS Poses Serious Risks,' *Wall Street Journal*, 15 April, at A13.
Institute of Medicine. 1988. *The Future of Public Health* (Washington, D.C.: National Academy Press).
Institute of Medicine. 1992. *Emerging Infections: Microbial Threats to Health in the United States* (Washington, D.C.: National Academy Press).
Institute of Medicine. 1997. *America's Vital Interest in Global Health* (Washington, D.C.: National Academy Press).
Institute of Medicine. 2003. *Microbial Threats to Health: Emergence, Detection, and Response*. Mark S. Smolinski, Margaret A. Hamburg, and Joshua Lederberg, eds (Washington, D.C.: National Academy Press).
International Covenant on Economic, Social, and Cultural Rights (ICESCR). 1966. In: Ian Brownlie, ed., *Basic Documents in International Law*, 4th edn (Oxford: Oxford University, 1995), pp. 263–75.
International Health Agency Act Hearings. 1971. Hearings before the Subcommittee on International Organizations and Movements of the Committee on Foreign Affairs, House of Representatives, 92nd Congress, 1st Session on H.R. 10042.
International Health Regulations. 1969. In: WHO, *International Health Regulations*, 3rd ann. edn (Geneva: WHO, 1983).
International Law Commission. 2001. *Draft Articles on Responsibility of States for Internationally Wrongful Acts*. UN General Assembly Resolution A/RES/56/83, 28 January.
International Sanitary Regulations. 1951. *World Health Organization: Technical Report Series, No. 41* (Geneva: WHO, 1951).
Jackson, R. 2001. 'The Evolution of International Society.' In: J. Baylis and S. Smith, eds, *The Globalization of World Politics: An Introduction to International Relations*, 2nd edn (Oxford: Oxford University Press), pp. 35–50.
Jakes, S. 2003. 'Beijing Hoodwinks WHO Inspectors,' *Time*, 18 April, at www.time.com/time/asia/news/printout/0,9788,444684,00.html.
Kant, I. 1795. *Eternal Peace and Other International Essays* (Boston: The World Peace Foundation, 1914).
Kapp, C. 2002. 'Global Fund Faces Uncertain Future as Cash Runs Low,' *The Lancet*; 360: 1225.
Kassalow, J. *Why Health is Important to U.S. Foreign Policy*, at www.milbank.org/reports/Foreignpolicy.html.
Kaul, I., Grunberg, I., and Stern, M.A., eds, 1999a. *Global Public Goods: International Cooperation in the 21st Century* (Oxford: Oxford University Press).

Kaul, I., Grunberg, I., and Stern, M.A. 1999b. 'Defining Global Public Goods.' In: I. Kaul, I. Grunberg, and M.A. Stern, eds, *Global Public Goods: International Cooperation in the 21st Century* (Oxford: Oxford University Press), pp. 2–19.

Kickbusch, I. 2002. 'Influence and Opportunity: Reflections on the U.S. Role in Global Public Health,' *Health Affairs*; 21: 131–41.

Kickbusch, I. 2003. 'Global Health Governance: Some Theoretical Considerations on the New Political Space.' In: K. Lee, ed., *Health Impacts of Globalization: Towards Global Governance* (Basingstoke: Palgrave Macmillan, 2003), pp. 192–203.

Klausner, R.D. *et al.* 2003. 'The Need for a Global HIV Vaccine Enterprise,' *Science*; 300: 2036–9.

Ksiazek, T.G. *et al.* 2003. 'A Novel Coronavirus Associated with Severe Acute Respiratory Syndrome,' *New England Journal of Medicine*; 348: 1953–66.

Lanord, C. 2002. *A Study of WHO's Official Relations System with Nongovernmental Organizations*. WHO Doc. CSI/2002/WP4.

Lee, K. and Dodgson, R. 2003. 'Globalization and Cholera: Implications for Global Governance.' In: K. Lee, ed., *Health Impacts of Globalization: Towards Global Governance* (Basingstoke: Palgrave Macmillan, 2003), pp. 123–43.

Legro, J. and Moravcsik, A. 1999. 'Is Anybody Still a Realist?,' *International Security*; 24: 5–55.

Leive, D.M. 1976. *International Regulatory Regimes: Case Studies in Health, Meterology, and Food*, Vol. I (Lexington, MA: Lexington Books).

Loughlin, K. and Berridge, V. 2002. *Global Health Governance: Historical Dimensions of Global Governance* (Discussion Paper No. 2) (London: Centre for Global Change and Health and WHO).

Mann, J.M. 1999. 'Human Rights and AIDS: The Future of the Pandemic.' In: J.M. Mann, S. Gruskin, M.A. Grodin, and G.J. Annas, eds, *Health and Human Rights: A Reader* (London: Routledge, 1999), pp. 216–26.

McClesky, E. 1996. 'Gore Unveils New Initiative for Fighting Infectious Diseases,' *BNA Health Care Daily*, 13 June, at LEXIS, Nexis Library, Curnws File.

McNeil, D.G. 2003. 'Health Officials Wield a Big Stick, Carefully, Against SARS,' *New York Times*, 20 April, at A12.

Médecins Sans Frontières Access to Essential Medicines Campaign and the Drugs for Neglected Diseases Working Group. 2001. *Fatal Imbalance: The Crisis in Research and Development for Drugs for Neglected Diseases* (Geneva: MSF and DND).

Médecins Sans Frontières. 2003a. *Positive Replication: A Médecins Sans Frontières* (MSF) *Background Paper for the 2nd IAS Conference on Pathogenesis and Treatment*, Paris, 13–16 July, at www.accessmed-msf.org/documents/englishiasdoc.pdf.

Médecins Sans Frontières. 2003b. *G-8 Offers World an 'Inaction' Plan on Health*, 9 June, at www.accessmed-msf.org/prod/publications.asp? scntid=3620031159124 &contenttype +PARA&.

Mirsky, J. 'How the Chinese Spread SARS,' *New York Review of Books*, 29 May.

Mooney, G. and Dzator, J. 2003. 'Global Public Goods for Health: A Flawed Paradigm?.' In: R.D. Smith, R. Beaglhole, D. Woodward, and N. Drager, eds, *Global Public Goods for Health: Health Economic and Public Health Perspectives* (Oxford: Oxford University Press, 2003), pp. 233–45.

Nakashima, E. 2003a. 'Vietnamese Cautiously Hail Progress on SARS; Strict Measures Planned to Prevent New Cases,' *Washington Post*, 1 May, at A11.

Nakashima, E. 2003b. 'Vietnam Took Lead in Containing SARS; Decisiveness, Luck Credited,' *Washington Post*, 5 May, at A01.

Narasimhan, V. and Attaran, A. 2003. 'Roll Back Malaria? The Scarcity of International Aid for Malaria Control,' *Malaria Journal*, at http://www.malaria-journal.com/content/2/1/8.

National Advisory Committee. 2003. *Learning from SARS: Renewal of Public Health in Canada – A Report of the National Advisory Committee on SARS and Public Health* (Ottawa: Health Canada).

National Intelligence Council. 2000. *The Global Infectious Disease Threat and Its Implications for the United States*. National Intelligence Estimate 99–17D, at www.cia.gov/cia/publications/nic/report/nie99-17d.html.

National Intelligence Council. 2003. *SARS: Down But Still a Threat*. Intelligence Community Assessment 2003–09.

National Science and Technology Council Committee on International Science, Engineering, and Technology (CISET) Working Group on Emerging and Re-Emerging Infectious Diseases. 1995. *Infectious Diseases – A Global Health Threat* (Washington, D.C.: CISET).

National Security Strategy of the United States of America. 2002 (Washington, D.C.: The White House).

Nussbaum, A. 1954. *A Concise History of the Law of Nations*, rev. edn (New York: Macmillan).

Office International de l'Hygiène Publique. 1907. Rome Agreement Establishing the International Office of Public Health, 9 December 1907. In: N.M. Goodman, *International Health Organizations and Their Work*, 2nd edn (London: Churchill Livingstone, 1971), pp. 101–4.

Pan, P.P. 2002. 'China Detaining Prominent AIDS Activist,' *Washington Post*, 7 September, at A14.

Pan, P.P. 2003. 'China Meets AIDS Crisis with Force,' *Washington Post*, 18 August, at A01.

Pan American Sanitary Bureau. 1902. *A History of the Pan American Health Organization* (Washington, D.C.: PAHO, 1992).

Pannenborg, C.O. 1979. *A New International Health Order: An Inquiry into the International Relations of World Health and Medical Care* (Alphen aan den Rijn: Sijthoff & Noordhoff).

Pei, M. 2003. *Remarks at Panel on China and SARS: The Crisis and Its Effects on Politics and the Economy*, 2 July.

Piller, C. 2003. 'In SARS Aftermath, the WHO's in Charge,' *Los Angeles Times*, 13 July, at A1.

Pomfret, J. 2003a. 'Hong Kong Official Takes Ill; Mystery Disease is Chief Suspect,' *Washington Post*, 25 March, at A06.

Pomfret, J. 2003b. 'China Raises Disease's Death Toll; Under Pressure, Officials Admit Spread of Infection to Beijing,' *Washington Post*, 27 March, at A16.

Pomfret, J. 2003c. 'Disease Forces Hong Kong School Closure; Officials Order Quarantine for 1,080 People to Combat Deadly Lung Ailment,' *Washington Post*, 28 March, at A19.

Pomfret, J. 2003d. 'China Agrees to Release Daily Reports on Disease,' *Washington Post*, 29 March, at A09.

Pomfret, J. 2003e. 'Respiratory Disease Spreads in Hong Kong,' *Washington Post*, 1 April, at A12.

Pomfret, J. 2003f. 'China Says Disease is in Check; Health Minister Encourages Tourism Despite WHO Advisory,' *Washington Post*, 4 April, at A15.

Pomfret, J. 2003g. 'Official Says China Erred on Outbreak; Rare Apology Cites "Poor Coordination,"' *Washington Post*, 5 April, at A14.
Pomfret, J. 2003h. 'China Says Finn Died of SARS; U.N. Official is First Foreigner to Succumb to Disease,' *Washington Post*, 7 April, at A08.
Pomfret, J. 2003i. 'Doctor Says Health Ministry Lied About Disease; Chinese Military Physician Accuses Beijing of Hiding Extent of Outbreak to Promote Tourism,' *Washington Post*, 10 April, at A26.
Pomfret, J. 2003j. 'As 10 More Die, Chinese Official Terms SARS 'Grave' Crisis; Premier Says Disease Outbreak Could Affect Nation's Stability,' *Washington Post*, 15 April, at A20.
Pomfret, J. 2003k. 'Beijing Said to Conceal Extent of Disease; Officials Try to Protect City's Reputation as World Health Agency Widens Probe,' *Washington Post*, 16 April, at A18.
Pomfret, J. 2003l. 'Underreporting, Secrecy Fuel SARS in Beijing, WHO Says,' *Washington Post*, 17 April, at A16.
Pomfret, J. 2003m. 'China Orders End to SARS Coverup; Officials Begin Belated Campaign Against Disease,' *Washington Post*, 19 April, at A08.
Pomfret, J. 2003n. 'Beijing Doctors Told to Hide SARS Victims,' *Washington Post*, 20 April, at A10.
Pomfret, J. 2003o. 'SARS Coverup Spurs a Shake-Up in Beijing,' *Washington Post*, 21 April, at A01.
Pomfret, J. 2003p. 'Epidemic is a "Test" for China's Leadership,' *Washington Post*, 22 April, at A15.
Pomfret, J. 2003q. 'China Broadens Effort Against SARS,' *Washington Post*, 28 April, at A01.
Pomfret, J. 2003r. 'Outbreak Gave China's Hu an Opening; President Responded to Pressure Inside and Outside Country on SARS,' *Washington Post*, 13 May, at A01.
Pomfret, J. 2003s. 'China Orders Officials to Give Full SARS Data,' *Washington Post*, 14 May, at A16.
Pomfret, J. 2003t. 'China Orders Halt to Debate on Reforms,' *Washington Post*, 27 August, at A01.
Pomfret, J. and Goodman, P.S. 2003. 'Mysterious Illness Kills 2 in Beijing in Sign of Spread,' *Washington Post*, 22 March, at A03.
Pomfret, J. and Weiss, R. 2003. 'Hong Kong Quarantines Complex to Control Spread of Epidemic,' *Washington Post*, 31 March, at A02.
Porter, D. 1999. *Health, Civilization, and the State* (London: Routledge).
Pottinger, M. 2003a. 'Hong Kong Hotel was a Virus Hub,' *Wall Street Journal*, 21 March, at B2.
Pottinger, M. 2003b. 'Asian Virus Transmitted to Others on Airplane,' *Wall Street Journal*, 26 March, at D2.
Pottinger, M. 2003c. 'Outraged Surgeon Forces China to Take a Dose of the Truth,' *Wall Street Journal*, 22 April, at A1.
Pottinger, M. 2003d. 'The SARS Outbreak: In Some Nations SARS Appears to Have Peaked,' *Wall Street Journal*, 29 April, at A2.
Pottinger, M. and Buckman, R. 2003. 'Holding Their Breath: A Mystery Illness Spreads in Asia, And So Does Fear,' *Wall Street Journal*, 28 March, at A1.
Pottinger, M. and Hutzler, C. 2003. 'New Ideas on SARS Emerge, and Doctor Questions Chinese Data,' *Wall Street Journal*, 9 April, at A10.

Pottinger, M., Regalado, A., and Cohen, M. 2003. 'Officials Alarmed by Spread of Respiratory Illness,' *Wall Street Journal*, 17 March, at A3.
ProMED. 2003. *About ProMED-mail*, at http://www.promedmail.org/pls/askus/f?p=2400:1950:5170440278578263877.
ProMED-mail. 2003. *Pneumonia—China (Guangdong): RFI*, 10 February, Archive Number 20030210.0357.
Price-Smith, A.T. 2002. *The Health of Nations: Infectious Disease, Environmental Change, and Their Effects on National Security and Development* (Cambridge, MA: MIT Press).
Regalado, A. and Dean, J. 2003. 'The SARS Outbreak: Hospital Lockdown in Taiwan Appears to Have Failed; Virus Has Spread Rapidly, Prompting U.S. Warning,' *Wall Street Journal*, 2 May, at B5.
Reich, M., ed. 2002. *Public–Private Partnerships for Health* (Cambridge, MA: Harvard University Press).
Reuters. 2003. 'WHO Predicts World Will Be Free of Human SARS Cases in a Few Weeks,' 27 June, at www.medscape.com/viewarticle/457998.
Richburg, K. 2003. 'Anxiety Spreading Faster than SARS; Alarm Common Even Where Disease Isn't,' *Washington Post*, 29 April, at A18.
Roelsgaard, E. 1974. 'Health Regulations and International Travel,' *Chronicle of the World Health Organization*; 28: 265–8.
Rosen, G. 1958. *A History of Public Health* (New York: MD Publications).
Rousseau, J.-J. 1756. 'Abstract and Judgement of Saint-Pierre's Project for Perpetual Peace.' In: S. Hoffmann and D.P. Fidler, eds, *Rousseau on International Relations* (Oxford: Clarendon Press, 1991), pp. 53–100.
Saich, A. 2003. 'The Real Fallout from China's Chernobyl,' *Financial Times*, 28 May, at 15.
SARS Expert Committee. 2003. *SARS in Hong Kong: From Experience to Action* (Hong Kong: SARS Expert Committee).
'SARS: Race to Patent Virus Renews Debate Over "Patents on Life,"' *Medical Letter on the CDC & FDA*, 1 June, at 2003 WestLaw 8982543.
Saywell, T. 2003. '"Superspreaders" Theory is Debated,' *Wall Street Journal*, 10 April, at D3.
Schacter, O. 1991. 'The Emergence of International Environmental Law,' *Journal of International Affairs*; 44: 457–93.
Scholte, J.A. 2000. *Globalization: A Critical Introduction* (Basingstoke: Palgrave – now Palgrave Macmillan).
Scholte, J.A. 2001. 'The Globalization of World Politics.' In: J. Baylis and S. Smith, eds, *The Globalization of World Politics: An Introduction to International Relations*, 2nd edn (Oxford: Oxford University Press), pp. 13–32.
Sharp, W.R. 1947. 'The New World Health Organization,' *American Journal of International Law*; 41: 509–29.
Shubber, S. 2000. *The International Code of Marketing of Breast-Milk Substitutes: An International Measure to Protect and Promote Breast-Feeding* (The Hague: Kluwer).
Siracusa Principles on the Limitations and Derogation Provisions in the International Covenant on Civil and Political Rights. 1985. UN Doc. E/CN.4/1985/4, Annex.
Slack, P. 1992. 'Introduction.' In: T. Ranger and P. Slack, eds, *Epidemics and Ideas: Essays on the Historical Perception of Pestilence* (Cambridge: Cambridge University Press), pp. 1–20.

Smith, R. and Woodward, D. 2003. 'Global Public Goods for Health: Use and Limitations.' In: R.D. Smith, R. Beaglehole, D. Woodward, and N. Drager, eds, *Global Public Goods for Health: Health Economic and Public Health Perspectives* (Oxford: Oxford University Press, 2003), pp. 246–65.

SS Lotus (France v. *Turkey)*. 1927. Permanent Court of International Justice, Series A, No. 10, *reprinted in* A. D'Amato, ed., *International Law Coursebook* (Cincinnati: Anderson Publishing, 1994), pp. 67–77.

Stein, R. 2003a. 'More Possible Cases of Respiratory Illness Investigated,' *Washington Post*, 18 March, at A24.

Stein, R. 2003b. 'Tests Suggest Virus Link; Lab Samples from 2 Outbreak Victims Show Signs of Microbe,' *Washington Post*, 19 March, at A09.

Stein, R. 2003c. 'Mystery Illness's Mortality Rate 4%, WHO Official Says,' *Washington Post*, 27 March, at A15.

Stein, R. 2003d. 'The Mystery Virus: A Guide to Origins, Symptoms and Precautions You Can Take,' *Washington Post*, 29 March, at A08.

Stein, R. 2003e. 'At CDC, Big Steps to Stem Epidemic; Warnings Cover Travel, Treatment,' *Washington Post*, 30 March, at A09.

Stein, R. 2003f. 'Epidemic Kills Scientist Who Helped Discover It,' *Washington Post*, 30 March, at A01.

Stein, R. 2003g. 'SARS Could Recur Anywhere at Any Time; Officials Warn of Virus's Ongoing Threat,' *Washington Post*, 1 May, at A11.

Stein, R. 2003h. 'SARS Epidemic is Over in Most of the World, Experts Say,' *Washington Post*, 18 May, at A12.

Stein, R. 2003i. 'Governments Can Control SARS, WHO Officials Say; International Spread Still a Concern,' *Washington Post*, 21 May, at A16.

Stein, R. 2003j. 'No New Deaths Reported for 1st Time in 2 Months,' *Washington Post*, 5 June, at A23.

Stein, R. and Brown, D. 2003. 'Illness May Have Spread on Plane; Respiratory Infection of Chinese Tourists Would be 1st Transmission on Flight,' *Washington Post*, 26 March, at A10.

Strange, S. 1995. 'Political Economy and International Relations.' In: K. Booth and S. Smith, eds, *International Relations Theory Today* (University Park, PA: Pennsylvania State University Press, 1995), pp. 154–74.

Taylor, A., Bettcher, D.W., and Peck, R. 2003. 'International Law and the International Legislative Process: The WHO Framework Convention on Tobacco Control.' In: R. Smith, R. Beaglehole, D. Woodward, and N. Drager, eds, *Global Public Goods for Health: Health Economic and Public Health Perspectives* (Oxford: Oxford University Press, 2003), pp. 212–29.

Tomasevski, K. 1995. 'Health.' In: O. Schachter and C.C. Joyner, eds, *United Nations Legal Order*, Vol. 2 (Cambridge: Cambridge University Press, 1995), pp. 859–906.

UNAIDS. 2002a. *AIDS Epidemic Update: December 2002* (Geneva: UNAIDS).

UNAIDS. 2002b. *Report on the Global HIV/AIDS Epidemic 2002* (Geneva: UNAIDS).

UNAIDS. 2002c. *HIV/AIDS: China's Titanic Peril* (Geneva: UNAIDS).

United Nations Charter. 1945. In: I. Brownlie, ed., *Basic Documents in International Law*, 4th edn (Oxford: Oxford University Press, 1995), pp. 1–35.

US Centers for Disease Control and Prevention. 1994. *Addressing Emerging Infectious Disease Threats: A Prevention Strategy for the United States* (Washington, D.C.: Department of Health and Human Services).

US Centers for Disease Control and Prevention. 2003. *Questions and Answers: Travel and Quarantine*, at www.cdc.gov/cidod/sars/qa/travel.htm.
US Department of State. 1947. 'International Health Security in the Modern World: The Sanitary Conventions and the World Health Organization,' *Department of State Bulletin*; 17: 953–8
US Public Health Service Act. 2003. 42 United States Code §264.
Velimirovic, B. 1976. 'Do We Still Need the International Health Regulations?,' *Journal of Infectious Diseases*; 133: 478–82.
Vienna Convention on the Law of Treaties. 1969. In: I. Brownlie, ed, *Basic Documents in International Law*, 4th edn (Oxford: Oxford University Press, 1995), pp. 388–425.
Vignes, C.-H. 1989. 'The Future of International Health Law: WHO Perspectives,' *International Digest of Health Legislation*; 40: 16–19.
Vincent, J. 1986. *Human Rights and International Relations* (Cambridge: Cambridge University Press).
Wall Street Journal. 2003a. 'Beijing Authorities Grant Slow Access to WHO Team,' *Wall Street Journal*, 14 April, at A17.
Wall Street Journal. 2003b. 'China's Other Disease,' *Wall Street Journal*, 22 April, at A28.
Waltz, K. 1979. *Theory of International Politics* (Reading, MA: Addison-Wesley).
Washington Post. 2002. 'Editorial – China Under Cover,' *Washington Post*, 2 September, at A22.
Washington Post. 2003a. 'Editorial – Fighting a Mystery Illness,' *Washington Post*, 2 April, at A16.
Washington Post. 2003b. 'Editorial – China's Chernobyl,' *Washington Post*, 22 April, at A18.
Watts, J. 2003. 'China Takes Drastic Action Over SARS Threat,' *The Lancet*; 361: 1708–9.
Widdus, R. 2001. 'Public–Private Partnerships for Health: Their Main Targets, Their Diversity, and Future Directions,' *Bulletin of the World Health Organization*; 79: 713–20.
Willetts, P. 2001. 'Transnational Actors and International Organizations in Global Politics.' In: J. Baylis and S. Smith, eds, *The Globalization of World Politics: An Introduction to International Relations*, 2nd edn (Oxford: Oxford University Press, 2001), pp. 356–83.
Winslow, C.-E. A. 1943. *The Conquest of Epidemic Disease: A Chapter in the History of Ideas* (Princeton: Princeton University Press).
Wonacott, P., Borsuk, R., and Cohen, M. 2003. 'Nations Step Up Efforts to Contain Deadly Ailment,' *Wall Street Journal*, 27 March, at D3.
Wonacott, P., Lawrence, S., and Pottinger, M. 2003. 'Health Officials Express Doubts About China's SARS Figures,' *Wall Street Journal*, 17 April, at D3.
Wonacott, P., McKay, B., and Hamilton, D.P. 2003. 'Fear of SARS Rises as Cases and Rumors Spread,' *Wall Street Journal*, 2 April, at B1.
Woodall, J. 1997. 'Outbreak Meets the Internet: Global Epidemic Monitoring by ProMED-mail,' *SIM Quarterly: Newsletter of the Society for the Internet in Medicine*, June.
Woodward, D. and Smith, R.D. 2003. 'Global Public Goods and Health: Concepts and Issues.' In: R.D. Smith, R. Beaglehole, D. Woodward, and N. Drager, eds, *Global Public Goods for Health: Health Economic and Public Health Perspectives* (Oxford: Oxford University Press, 2003), pp. 3–29.

World Bank. 1993. *World Development Report 1993: Investing In Health* (Washington, D.C.: World Bank).
World Health Assembly. 1995. *Revision and Updating of the International Health Regulations*. WHA48.7, 12 May.
World Health Assembly. 2001. *Global Health Security: Epidemic Alert and Response*, WHA54.14, 21 May.
World Health Assembly. 2003a. *Severe Acute Respiratory Syndrome (SARS)*. WHA56.29, 28 May.
World Health Assembly. 2003b. *Revision of the International Health Regulations*. WHA56.28, 28 May.
WHO. 1948. 'Constitution of the WHO.' In: WHO, *Basic Documents*, 40th edn (Geneva: WHO, 1994), pp. 1–18.
WHO. 1970. 'Cholera,' *Weekly Epidemiological Record*; 45: 377.
WHO. 1985. 'International Health Regulations (1969),' *Weekly Epidemiological Record*; 60: 311.
WHO. 1986. 'Functioning of the International Health Regulations for the Period from 1 January to 31 December 1985 (Part I) – Vaccination Certificate Requirements and Health Advice for International Travel,' *Weekly Epidemiological Record*; 61: 389.
WHO. 1988. 'Principles Governing Relations Between the World Health Organization and Nongovernmental Organizations.' In: WHO, *Basic Documents*, 40th edn (Geneva: WHO, 1994), pp. 74–9.
WHO. 1995. *The International Response to Epidemics and Applications of the International Health Regulations: Report of a WHO Informal Consultation*. WHO Doc. WHO/EMC/IHR/96.1, December 11–14.
WHO. 1996. *World Health Report: Fighting Disease, Fostering Development* (Geneva: WHO).
WHO. 1998. *Director-General Says Food Import Bans Are Inappropriate for Fighting Cholera*, Press Release WHO/24, 16 February.
WHO. 1999. *Removing Obstacles to Healthy Development* (Geneva: WHO).
WHO. 2002a. *Global Defence Against the Infectious Disease Threat*. Mary Kay Kindhauser, ed. (Geneva: WHO).
WHO. 2002b. Coordinates 2002 – Charting Progress Against AIDS, TB, and Malaria, at www.who.int/infectious-disease-news/.
WHO. 2002c. *World Health Report 2002: Reducing Risks, Promoting Healthy Life* (Geneva: WHO).
WHO. 2002d. *Global Crises – Global Solutions: Managing Public Health Emergencies of International Concern Through the Revised International Health Regulations* (Geneva: WHO).
WHO. 2003a. Cumulative Number of Reported Probable Cases of SARS, 7 August, at www.who.int/csr/sars/country/2003_08_07/en.html.
WHO. 2003b. *Severe Acute Respiratory Syndrome (SARS): Status of the Outbreak and Lessons for the Immediate Future* (Geneva: WHO).
WHO. 2003c. Acute Respiratory Syndrome in China, 11 February, at www.who.int/csr/don/2003_02_11/en/.
WHO. 2003d. Acute Respiratory Syndrome in China – Update, 12 February, at www.who.int/csr/don/2003_02_12/en/.
WHO. 2003e. Acute Respiratory Syndrome in China – Update 2, 14 February, at www.who.int/csr/don/2003_02_14/en/.

WHO. 2003f. Influenza (H5N1) in Hong Kong Special Administrative Region of China, 19 February, at www.who.int/csr/don/2003_02_19/en/.
WHO. 2003g. Influenza (H5N1) in Hong Kong Special Administrative Region of China – Update, 20 February, at www.who.int/csr/don/2003_02_20/en/.
WHO. 2003h. Acute Respiratory Syndrome in China – Update 3, 20 February, at www.who.int/csr/don/2003_02_20/en/.
WHO. 2003i. Influenza (H5N1) in Hong Kong Special Administrative Region of China – Update 2, 27 February, at www.who.int/csr/don/2003_02_27a/en/.
WHO. 2003j. Acute Respiratory Syndrome in Hong Kong Special Administrative Region of China/Viet Nam, 12 March, at www.who.int/csr/don/2003_03_12/en/.
WHO. 2003k. Severe Acute Respiratory Syndrome (SARS) Multi-Country Outbreak, 15 March, at www.who.int/csr/don/2003_03_15/en/.
WHO. 2003l. Severe Acute Respiratory Syndrome (SARS) Multi-Country Outbreak – Update, 16 March, at www.who.int/csr/don/2003_03_16/en/.
WHO. 2003m. Severe Acute Respiratory Syndrome (SARS) Multi-Country Outbreak – Update 2, 17 March, at www.who.int/csr/don/2003_03_17/en/.
WHO. 2003n. Severe Acute Respiratory Syndrome (SARS) Multi-Country Outbreak – Update 3, 18 March, at www.who.int/csr/don/2003_03_18/en/.
WHO. 2003o. Severe Acute Respiratory Syndrome (SARS) Multi-Country Outbreak – Update 4, 19 March, at www.who.int/csr/don/2003_03_19/en/.
WHO. 2003p. Severe Acute Respiratory Syndrome (SARS) Multi-Country Outbreak – Update 5, 20 March, at www.who.int/csr/don/2003_03_20/en/.
WHO. 2003q. Severe Acute Respiratory Syndrome (SARS) Multi-Country Outbreak – Update 6, 21 March, at www.who.int/csr/don/2003_03_21/en/.
WHO. 2003r. Severe Acute Respiratory Syndrome (SARS) Multi-Country Outbreak – Update 7, 22 March, at www.who.int/csr/don/2003_03_22/en/.
WHO. 2003s. Severe Acute Respiratory Syndrome (SARS) Multi-Country Outbreak – Update 9, 25 March, at www.who.int/csr/don/2003_03_25/en/.
WHO. 2003t. Severe Acute Respiratory Syndrome (SARS) Multi-Country Outbreak – Update 10, 26 March, at www.who.int/csr/don/2003_03_26/en/.
WHO. 2003u. Severe Acute Respiratory Syndrome (SARS) Multi-Country Outbreak – Update 12, 27 March, at www.who.int/csr/don/2003_03_276/en/.
WHO. 2003v. Severe Acute Respiratory Syndrome (SARS) Multi-Country Outbreak – Update 13, 28 March, at www.who.int/csr/don/2003_03_28/en/.
WHO. 2003w. Severe Acute Respiratory Syndrome (SARS) Multi-Country Outbreak – Update 14, 29 March, at www.who.int/csr/don/2003_03_29/en/.
WHO. 2003x. Severe Acute Respiratory Syndrome (SARS) Multi-Country Outbreak – Update 15, 31 March, at www.who.int/csr/don/2003_03_31/en/.
WHO. 2003y. Severe Acute Respiratory Syndrome (SARS) Multi-Country Outbreak – Update 16, 1 April, at www.who.int/csr/don/2003_04_01/en/.
WHO. 2003z. Severe Acute Respiratory Syndrome (SARS) Multi-Country Outbreak – Update 17, 2 April, at www.who.int/csr/don/2003_04_02/en/.
WHO.2003a-1. Severe Acute Respiratory Syndrome (SARS) Multi-Country Outbreak – Update 18, 2 April, at www.who.int/csr/don/2003_04_02a/en/.
WHO.2003b-1. Severe Acute Respiratory Syndrome (SARS) Multi-Country Outbreak – Update 19, 2 April, at www.who.int/csr/don/2003_04_02b/en/.
WHO.2003c-1. Severe Acute Respiratory Syndrome (SARS) Multi-Country Outbreak – Update 21, 4 April, at www.who.int/csr/don/2003_04_04/en/.

WHO. 2003d-1. Severe Acute Respiratory Syndrome (SARS) Multi-Country Outbreak – Update 23, 7 April, at www.who.int/csr/don/2003_04_07/en/.
WHO. 2003e-1. Severe Acute Respiratory Syndrome (SARS) Multi-Country Outbreak – Update 24, 8 April, at www.who.int/csr/don/2003_04_08/en/.
WHO. 2003f-1. Severe Acute Respiratory Syndrome (SARS) Multi-Country Outbreak – Update 25, 9 April, at www.who.int/csr/don/2003_04_09/en/.
WHO. 2003g-1. Severe Acute Respiratory Syndrome (SARS) Multi-Country Outbreak – Update 27, 11 April, at www.who.int/csr/don/2003_04_11/en/.
WHO. 2003h-1. Severe Acute Respiratory Syndrome (SARS) Multi-Country Outbreak – Update 28, 12 April, at www.who.int/csr/don/2003_04_12/en/.
WHO. 2003i-1. Severe Acute Respiratory Syndrome (SARS) Multi-Country Outbreak – Update 29, 14 April, at www.who.int/csr/don/2003_04_14/en/.
WHO. 2003j-1. Severe Acute Respiratory Syndrome (SARS) Multi-Country Outbreak – Update 30, 15 April, at www.who.int/csr/don/2003_04_15/en/.
WHO. 2003k-1. Severe Acute Respiratory Syndrome (SARS) Multi-Country Outbreak – Update 31, 16 April, at www.who.int/csr/don/2003_04_16/en/.
WHO. 2003l-1. Severe Acute Respiratory Syndrome (SARS) Multi-Country Outbreak – Update 32, 17 April, at www.who.int/csr/don/2003_04_17/en/.
WHO. 2003m-1. Severe Acute Respiratory Syndrome (SARS) Multi-Country Outbreak – Update 33, 18 April, at www.who.int/csr/don/2003_04_18/en/.
WHO. 2003n-1. Severe Acute Respiratory Syndrome (SARS) Multi-Country Outbreak – Update 34, 19 April, at www.who.int/csr/don/2003_04_19/en/.
WHO. 2003o-1. Severe Acute Respiratory Syndrome (SARS) Multi-Country Outbreak – Update 35, 21 April, at www.who.int/csr/don/2003_04_21/en/
WHO. 2003p-1. Severe Acute Respiratory Syndrome (SARS) Multi-Country Outbreak – Update 37, 23 April, at www.who.int/csr/don/2003_04_23/en/.
WHO. 2003q-1. Severe Acute Respiratory Syndrome (SARS) Multi-Country Outbreak – Update 39, 25 April, at www.who.int/csr/don/2003_04_25/en/.
WHO. 2003r-1. Severe Acute Respiratory Syndrome (SARS) Multi-Country Outbreak – Update 41, 28 April, at www.who.int/csr/don/2003_04_28/en/.
WHO. 2003s-1. Severe Acute Respiratory Syndrome (SARS) Multi-Country Outbreak – Update 42, 29 April, at www.who.int/csr/don/2003_04_29/en/.
WHO. 2003t-1. Severe Acute Respiratory Syndrome (SARS) Multi-Country Outbreak – Update 43, 30 April, at www.who.int/csr/don/2003_04_30/en/.
WHO. 2003u-1. Severe Acute Respiratory Syndrome (SARS) Multi-Country Outbreak – Update 44, 1 May, at www.who.int/csr/don/2003_05_01/en/.
WHO. 2003v-1. Severe Acute Respiratory Syndrome (SARS) Multi-Country Outbreak – Update 46, 3 May, at www.who.int/csr/don/2003_05_03/en/.
WHO. 2003w-1. Severe Acute Respiratory Syndrome (SARS) Multi-Country Outbreak – Update 47, 5 May, at www.who.int/csr/don/2003_05_05/en/.
WHO. 2003x-1. Severe Acute Respiratory Syndrome (SARS) Multi-Country Outbreak – Update 49, 7 May, at www.who.int/csr/don/2003_05_07a/en/.
WHO. 2003y-1. Severe Acute Respiratory Syndrome (SARS) Multi-Country Outbreak – Update 50, 8 May, at www.who.int/csr/don/2003_05_08/en/.
WHO. 2003z-1. Severe Acute Respiratory Syndrome (SARS) Multi-Country Outbreak – Update 51, 9 May, at www.who.int/csr/don/2003_05_09/en/.
WHO. 2003a-2. Severe Acute Respiratory Syndrome (SARS) Multi-Country Outbreak – Update 54, 13 May, at www.who.int/csr/don/2003_05_13/en/.

WHO. 2003b-2. Severe Acute Respiratory Syndrome (SARS) Multi-Country Outbreak – Update 55, 14 May, at www.who.int/csr/don/2003_05_14/en/.

WHO. 2003c-2. Severe Acute Respiratory Syndrome (SARS) Multi-Country Outbreak – Update 57, 16 May, at www.who.int/csr/don/2003_05_16/en/.

WHO. 2003d-2. Severe Acute Respiratory Syndrome (SARS) Multi-Country Outbreak – Update 58, 17 May, at www.who.int/csr/don/2003_05_17/en/.

WHO. 2003e-2. Severe Acute Respiratory Syndrome (SARS) Multi-Country Outbreak – Update 59, 19 May, at www.who.int/csr/don/2003_05_19a/en/.

WHO. 2003f-2. Severe Acute Respiratory Syndrome (SARS) Multi-Country Outbreak – Update 60, 20 May, at www.who.int/csr/don/2003_05_20/en/.

WHO. 2003g-2. Severe Acute Respiratory Syndrome (SARS) Multi-Country Outbreak – Update 61, 21 May, at www.who.int/csr/don/2003_05_21a/en/.

WHO. 2003h-2. Severe Acute Respiratory Syndrome (SARS) Multi-Country Outbreak – Update 62, 22 May, at www.who.int/csr/don/2003_05_22/en/.

WHO. 2003i-2. Severe Acute Respiratory Syndrome (SARS) Multi-Country Outbreak – Update 63, 23 May, at www.who.int/csr/don/2003_05_23/en/.

WHO. 2003j-2. Severe Acute Respiratory Syndrome (SARS) Multi-Country Outbreak – Update 64, 23 May, at www.who.int/csr/don/2003_05_23b/en/.

WHO. 2003k-2. Severe Acute Respiratory Syndrome (SARS) Multi-Country Outbreak – Update 66, 26 May, at www.who.int/csr/don/2003_05_26/en/.

WHO. 2003l-2. Severe Acute Respiratory Syndrome (SARS) Multi-Country Outbreak – Update 68, 28 May, at www.who.int/csr/don/2003_05_28/en/.

WHO. 2003m-2. Severe Acute Respiratory Syndrome (SARS) Multi-Country Outbreak – Update 69, 29 May, at www.who.int/csr/don/2003_05_29/en/.

WHO. 2003n-2. Severe Acute Respiratory Syndrome (SARS) Multi-Country Outbreak – Update 70, 30 May, at www.who.int/csr/don/2003_05_30a/en/.

WHO. 2003o-2. Severe Acute Respiratory Syndrome (SARS) Multi-Country Outbreak – Update 73, 4 June, at www.who.int/csr/don/2003_06_04/en/.

WHO. 2003p-2. Severe Acute Respiratory Syndrome (SARS) Multi-Country Outbreak – Update 76, 9 June, at www.who.int/csr/don/2003_06_09/en/.

WHO. 2003q-2. Severe Acute Respiratory Syndrome (SARS) Multi-Country Outbreak – Update 77, 10 June, at www.who.int/csr/don/2003_06_10/en/.

WHO. 2003r-2. Severe Acute Respiratory Syndrome (SARS) Multi-Country Outbreak – Update 79, 12 June, at www.who.int/csr/don/2003_06_12/en/.

WHO. 2003s-2. Severe Acute Respiratory Syndrome (SARS) Multi-Country Outbreak – Update 80, 13 June, at www.who.int/csr/don/2003_06_13/en/.

WHO. 2003t-2. Severe Acute Respiratory Syndrome (SARS) Multi-Country Outbreak – Update 83, 18 June, at www.who.int/csr/don/2003_06_18/en/.

WHO. 2003u-2. Severe Acute Respiratory Syndrome (SARS) Multi-Country Outbreak – Update 84, 19 June, at www.who.int/csr/don/2003_06_19/en/.

WHO. 2003v-2. Severe Acute Respiratory Syndrome (SARS) Multi-Country Outbreak – Update 86, 23 June, at www.who.int/csr/don/2003_06_23/en/.

WHO. 2003w-2. Severe Acute Respiratory Syndrome (SARS) Multi-Country Outbreak – Update 87, 24 June, at www.who.int/csr/don/2003_06_24/en/.

WHO. 2003x-2. Severe Acute Respiratory Syndrome (SARS) Multi-Country Outbreak – Update 91, 30 June, at www.who.int/csr/don/2003_06_30/en/.

WHO. 2003y-2. Severe Acute Respiratory Syndrome (SARS) Multi-Country Outbreak – Update 92, 1 July, at www.who.int/csr/don/2003_07_01/en/.

WHO. 2003z-2. Severe Acute Respiratory Syndrome (SARS) Multi-Country Outbreak – Update 93, 2 July, at www.who.int/csr/don/2003_07_02/en/.

WHO. 2003a-3. Severe Acute Respiratory Syndrome (SARS) Multi-Country Outbreak – Update 96, 2 July, at www.who.int/csr/don/2003_07_05/en/.

WHO. 2003b-3. SARS Outbreak Contained Worldwide: Threat Remains and More Research Needed, Says WHO, 5 July, at www.who.int/mediacentre/releases/2003/pr56/en

WHO. 2003c-3. World Health Organization Announces New Public–Private Initiative on Disease Surveillance and Response, 22, May, at www.who.int/mediacentre/releases/2003/prwha3/en/.

WHO. 2003d-3. Disease Outbreaks – Archives by Disease, at www.who.int/disease-outbreak-news-disease/bydisease.htm.

WHO. 2003e-3. Alert, Verification and Public Health Management of SARS in the Post-Outbreak Period, at www.who.int/csr/sars/postoutbreak/en/.

WHO. 2003f-3. Influenza Vaccination for the 2003–04 Season: Recommendations in the Context of Concern About SARS, at www.who.int/csr/disease/influenza/sars/en/.

WHO. 2003g-3. *Metropole Hotel: Final Report of WHO Environmental Investigation* (unpublished document).

World Trade Organization. 2001. *Declaration on the TRIPS Agreement and Public Health,* at www.wto.org/english/thewto_e/minist_e/min01_e/mindecl_trips_e.htm.

Xu, W. 2003. 'What Will it Take to Transform China?,' *Washington Post,* 19 May, at A19.

Yach, D. and Bettcher, D. 1998. 'The Globalization of Public Health,' *American Journal of Public Health*; 88: 735–41.

Index